KATE HALE

Maternity Fashion and Comfort

Stylish and Practical Choices for Every Stage

Contents

Introduction

Pregnancy is a unique journey filled with excitement, anticipation, and undeniable physical and emotional changes. One of the most significant changes that expecting mothers experience is the transformation of their bodies. These changes are beautiful and essential but can also present challenges when it comes to feeling comfortable and confident in your clothes. Maternity fashion is more than just accommodating a growing belly; it's about creating a sense of style that evolves with you and allows you to embrace your new form while ensuring you feel as comfortable as possible.

This book, *Maternity Fashion and Comfort: Stylish and Practical Choices for Every Stage,* is designed to guide you through each stage of your pregnancy journey, helping you strike the perfect balance between comfort and style. It's not just about what you wear; it's about how you feel in your clothes and how your wardrobe can support both your physical needs and emotional well-being.

In this introduction, we will explore the importance of maternity fashion and comfort, address how to navigate the changes that come with pregnancy, and offer insight into how to use this book to make practical, stylish choices at every stage of pregnancy.

The Journey to Motherhood: Embracing Your Changing Body

The journey to motherhood is a trans-formative experience that affects every part of your life, including your relationship with your body. From the early stages of pregnancy to the postpartum period, your body will go through a series of changes that can be both exciting and overwhelming. As your baby grows, your body adapts to accommodate the new life forming inside of you. With these changes come new needs, especially when it comes to fashion.

1. Physical Changes Throughout Pregnancy

During pregnancy, your body undergoes a variety of changes that can impact how you feel and how your clothes fit. In the first trimester, you may experience bloating and slight changes in your waistline, but it's often subtle enough that your regular clothes may still fit. As you move into the second trimester, your baby bump becomes more pronounced, and your body begins to store more fat to support your growing baby. By the third trimester, your body is fully preparing for childbirth, and your clothing needs become even more specific as you seek more room, flexibility, and support.

These changes can make dressing yourself a challenge, especially if you're trying to maintain a sense of style. Finding clothes that fit, flatter, and feel comfortable becomes a priority. Maternity fashion is designed specifically with these changes in mind, offering solutions that adapt to your growing body and keep you comfortable while still allowing you to express your personal style.

2. Emotional and Psychological Shifts

Along with the physical changes, pregnancy often brings emotional and psychological shifts that can influence how you feel about your body and how you dress. For many women, there's a tension between celebrating their pregnancy and grappling with the challenges that come with body changes. You may have days where you feel empowered by the life growing inside of you and other days where you struggle with body image issues.

It's important to embrace these changes as part of the beautiful, natural process of becoming a mother. Maternity fashion plays a significant role in this by providing options that allow you to feel good about yourself, no matter what stage you're in. Clothing that fits well, feels good on your skin, and flatters your changing shape can boost your confidence and help you maintain a positive relationship with your body during this trans-formative time.

3. Embracing the Beauty of Change

One of the key messages this book aims to impart is the importance of embracing the changes your body undergoes during pregnancy. Instead of resisting these changes or feeling frustrated by them, maternity fashion allows you to work with your body, dressing in a way that enhances your natural beauty and supports your physical needs. This is a time to celebrate the strength and resilience of your body as it nurtures new life.

Maternity fashion offers a range of solutions that cater to different stages of pregnancy and body types. From stretchy, breathable fabrics to designs that grow with you, the focus is on providing clothes that make you feel beautiful and comfortable. Whether you're lounging at home, going to work, or attending a special event, the right maternity outfit can make all the difference in how you feel.

The Balance Between Style and Comfort

One of the biggest challenges of maternity fashion is finding the right balance between style and comfort. As your body changes, comfort becomes paramount, but that doesn't mean you have to sacrifice style. The idea that maternity clothes are all about oversize, shapeless garments is outdated. Today's maternity fashion is as much about aesthetics as it is about practicality.

1. Comfort is Key

Pregnancy comes with physical discomforts, from back pain to swollen feet, and the last thing you need is for your clothes to add to that discomfort.

Prioritizing comfort means choosing fabrics that are soft, stretchy, and breathable. Cotton, bamboo, and modal are all great options for maternity clothes because they provide comfort without restricting movement. These fabrics also allow your skin to breathe, reducing irritation and helping to keep you cool.

Design features like adjustable waistbands, stretchy panels, and ruching are staples of modern maternity fashion. These details ensure that your clothes grow with you, offering support and flexibility as your belly expands. Comfort isn't just about the physical fit, though—it's also about feeling at ease in your own skin, and the right clothes can help with that. Well-fitting maternity clothing that flatters your figure can boost your confidence and make you feel more comfortable in your changing body.

2. Maintaining Your Personal Style

For many women, pregnancy can feel like a time when their personal style is put on hold. However, maternity fashion has come a long way in offering stylish options that allow you to maintain your sense of self while accommodating your growing body. You don't have to give up your favorite looks just because you're pregnant—whether you prefer minimalist chic, bold patterns, or timeless classics, there are maternity options that fit every aesthetic.

Maintaining your personal style during pregnancy is important because it helps you feel like yourself. Fashion is a form of self-expression, and just because your body is changing doesn't mean you have to abandon that part of yourself. In fact, pregnancy can be an opportunity to experiment with new styles, discover new trends, and find fresh ways to express yourself through fashion.

3. Finding Versatile Pieces

One of the keys to balancing style and comfort is finding versatile maternity pieces that can be dressed up or down and worn throughout different stages of your pregnancy. For example, a well-made pair of maternity jeans with a stretchy waistband can be paired with a casual t-shirt for everyday wear or dressed up with a blouse and blazer for a more polished look. Maternity dresses are another versatile option—they're comfortable, easy to wear, and can be styled for both casual and formal occasions.

Layering is another great way to add versatility to your maternity wardrobe. Lightweight cardigans, scarves, and jackets can be worn over maternity basics to create different looks without sacrificing comfort. Investing in a few key pieces that you can mix and match will allow you to create a variety of outfits without needing an entirely new wardrobe.

4. Accessories to Elevate Your Look

Accessories play a big role in maternity fashion. Since your body is constantly changing, you may find that certain clothing items fit differently from week to week. Accessories like scarves, belts, and jewelry can help add a personal touch to your outfits, allowing you to feel more put together even on days when comfort is your top priority.

Belts are particularly useful during pregnancy because they can help define your waist and create a more tailored look, especially with looser dresses or tunics. Scarves and shawls are also great options because they add both style and practicality, providing warmth without the bulk of heavy layers. A well-chosen piece of jewelry can draw attention to your best features and complement your overall look, adding a touch of sophistication or fun to your outfit.

How to Use This Book for Every Stage of Pregnancy

This book is designed to be a comprehensive guide to maternity fashion and comfort, taking you through each stage of pregnancy with practical advice, styling tips, and solutions for common fashion dilemmas. No matter where you are in your pregnancy journey, you'll find valuable information to help you dress comfortably and stylishly.

1. First Trimester: Transitioning Your Wardrobe

In the first trimester, many women can still wear their regular clothes, but you may start to notice changes in your waistline or bust. This is a great time to begin transitioning your wardrobe by investing in a few key pieces that will grow with you. Stretchy leggings, flowy tops, and adjustable bras are great options for this stage. The book will offer advice on how to make the most of your current wardrobe while preparing for the changes ahead.

2. Second Trimester: Embracing Maternity Fashion

The second trimester is often when the baby bump becomes more noticeable, and you may find that your regular clothes no longer fit as comfortably. This is the time to start embracing maternity fashion and investing in pieces specifically designed for pregnancy. From maternity jeans to dresses that flatter your growing bump, this book will guide you in finding clothes that make you feel good while accommodating your changing body.

3. Third Trimester: Prioritizing Comfort

In the third trimester, comfort becomes even more important as your body reaches its peak size and you prepare for childbirth. You'll need clothes that are not only comfortable but also provide support. The book will help you find solutions for common third-trimester issues like swollen feet, back pain, and finding clothes that fit over your bump. Loose-fitting dresses, supportive bras, and maternity Lounge-wear are essential during this stage.

4. Postpartum: Transitioning Back to Your Pre-Pregnancy Wardrobe

After giving birth, your body will continue to change as you recover and adjust to life with a newborn. The postpartum period is a time of healing and adjustment, and your wardrobe should reflect that. You may not immediately return to your pre-pregnancy body, and that's completely normal. In fact, many women find that they need to wear maternity clothes for a few months after giving birth. This book will guide you through this transitional period, offering tips on how to gradually shift back to your pre-pregnancy wardrobe while incorporating postpartum-friendly pieces, like nursing tops, comfortable Lounge-wear, and loose-fitting dresses.

Creating a Postpartum Wardrobe

After giving birth, your body will continue to go through changes as it recovers from childbirth. One of the first things to keep in mind is comfort—your body will need time to heal, so it's important to wear clothes that support this process. Loose-fitting clothing, soft fabrics, and nursing-friendly options are all essential during this time.

Many women also experience postpartum swelling and discomfort, so opting for clothes with stretch and flexibility is key. Nursing bras, wrap dresses, and button-down tops make breastfeeding easier, while maternity leggings and joggers provide comfort for daily activities or lounging at home.

1. Adapting Your Maternity Clothes Postpartum

One of the most economical and practical approaches to dressing postpartum is continuing to wear some of your maternity clothes. Items like maternity leggings, maxi dresses, and stretchy tops are still comfortable and functional for postpartum wear. These pieces are often designed with flexibility in mind, which is perfect for the postpartum phase when your body is still changing.

Additionally, nursing-friendly options like button-down shirts or dresses with easy access to breastfeeding can serve double duty. Clothes with an adjustable fit, like wrap tops or dresses, are great for transitioning between stages as your body slowly returns to its pre-pregnancy shape.

2. Gradually Reintroducing Your Pre-Pregnancy Clothes

While your body may not return to its pre-pregnancy size right away (or at all, in some cases), there are ways to slowly reintroduce items from your pre-pregnancy wardrobe. Loose-fitting pieces like cardigans, oversize shirts, and flowy skirts can work well during the postpartum phase. You may want to mix these items with your maternity wear to create a wardrobe that feels both familiar and comfortable. The book will offer tips on how to incorporate your favorite pieces back into your wardrobe without compromising on comfort or practicality.

The Role of Self-Care in Maternity Fashion

Throughout your pregnancy and postpartum journey, it's essential to prioritize self-care, and your wardrobe plays a crucial role in this. What you wear can significantly affect how you feel—both physically and emotionally. Choosing clothes that make you feel good about yourself is a form of self-care. The book emphasizes the importance of dressing in a way that supports your mental and emotional well-being, as well as your physical comfort.

During pregnancy, it's easy to feel disconnected from your body, especially as it undergoes so many changes. One way to maintain a sense of self during this time is by investing in pieces that reflect your personal style while accommodating your new body. When you feel good in your clothes, you're more likely to feel confident and empowered, which can help you embrace the changes that come with pregnancy.

Building a Long-Lasting Maternity Wardrobe

One of the goals of this book is to help you build a long-lasting maternity wardrobe that not only serves you during pregnancy but also adapts to your postpartum needs and beyond. A well-thought-out maternity wardrobe doesn't have to be extensive or expensive; it should be versatile, comfortable, and reflective of your personal style.

1. Investing in Quality Pieces

Instead of buying a large number of inexpensive maternity clothes, it's worth investing in a few quality pieces that will last throughout your pregnancy and beyond. High-quality fabrics and well-constructed garments will be more comfortable, durable, and adaptable as your body changes. This approach also allows you to build a wardrobe that you can rely on for future pregnancies or that you can pass on to others.

2. Versatility is Key

Versatility is the cornerstone of a functional maternity wardrobe. Many maternity clothes are designed to be worn throughout multiple stages of pregnancy and into the postpartum period. Items like stretchy dresses, adjustable waistbands, and nursing-friendly tops are perfect examples of versatile pieces that can be worn long after your baby is born. The book will guide you through choosing these adaptable pieces and suggest ways to style them for different occasions.

3. Minimalism Meets Practicality

There's no need to overhaul your entire wardrobe when you become pregnant. The concept of a capsule maternity wardrobe—a collection of essential, versatile pieces—allows you to create numerous outfits without needing an extensive wardrobe. You'll learn how to make the most of a small selection of well-chosen garments, mixing and matching them to create different looks that suit your lifestyle.

By focusing on quality over quantity, you'll not only save money but also ensure that every piece in your maternity wardrobe is practical and purposeful. This book will show you how to build a minimalist maternity wardrobe that works for all stages of pregnancy and beyond, offering styling tips, product recommendations, and practical advice.

Conclusion: Preparing for a Stylish and Comfortable Pregnancy

In this introduction, we've touched on the importance of maternity fashion and comfort, embracing the changes that come with pregnancy, and how this book can help guide you through every stage of the journey. From early pregnancy to postpartum recovery, maternity fashion is about much more than just finding clothes that fit—it's about feeling confident, comfortable, and connected to your body as it grows and changes.

This book is your go-to guide for navigating the world of maternity fashion, offering practical advice and style solutions that are both functional and fashionable. With each chapter, you'll gain new insights into how to dress for every stage of pregnancy, how to balance style with comfort, and how to build a wardrobe that supports your physical and emotional well-being.

Whether you're in the early stages of pregnancy or preparing for postpartum life, this book will equip you with the tools you need to feel empowered in your maternity journey. You'll learn how to adapt your wardrobe to meet your changing needs, how to maintain your personal style, and how to prioritize comfort without sacrificing fashion.

As you embark on this exciting journey to motherhood, remember that fashion is not just about what you wear—it's about how you feel. With the right maternity wardrobe, you can embrace the changes in your body with confidence and grace, knowing that you're dressed for comfort, style, and everything in between.

Understanding Your Changing Body

Pregnancy is an extraordinary journey that brings with it many physical, emotional, and psychological transformations. Your body will go through numerous changes across each trimester, and these changes not only affect how you feel but also how you dress. Understanding the way your body evolves during pregnancy is crucial to making informed decisions about your wardrobe, ensuring that you stay comfortable while maintaining a sense of style.

In this chapter, we will delve into the body changes you can expect in each trimester, the common wardrobe pitfalls to avoid, and how to adapt your pre-pregnancy wardrobe to accommodate your new shape. The key is to build a maternity wardrobe that grows with you, offering flexibility, comfort, and style at every stage.

Body Changes in Each Trimester

As your body goes through pregnancy, you will experience different changes in each trimester. These changes are part of the natural progression of pregnancy and, while they may sometimes feel overwhelming, understanding what to expect can make it easier to dress comfortably and confidently.

First Trimester: Subtle Beginnings

The first trimester, spanning from week 1 to week 12 of pregnancy, is often characterized by subtle bodily changes. For many women, the physical transformation during this stage is minimal, though some may experience bloating or slight weight gain. During these early weeks, your baby is still very small, and your uterus remains within the pelvic region, meaning that your bump will likely not be visible yet.

However, hormonal changes can cause significant shifts in how your body feels. You may experience tenderness in your breasts, morning sickness, and fatigue, all of which can influence how comfortable you feel in your clothes. While most women can continue wearing their regular clothes in the first trimester, some may need to make minor adjustments, such as opting for looser-fitting tops and bottoms to accommodate bloating.

Additionally, during this stage, some women may begin to notice changes in their bust size, as their bodies start preparing for breastfeeding. For this reason, it may be helpful to invest in comfortable, non-restrictive bras early on, as they will provide support without putting pressure on your sensitive breasts.

Dressing for the First Trimester

During the first trimester, comfort is key. You'll likely be able to wear much of your pre-pregnancy wardrobe, but it's important to pay attention to how your body feels. Consider choosing clothes that offer a bit more flexibility and comfort, especially in the waistline and chest area. Stretchy leggings, flowy blouses, and dresses that aren't too tight around the middle can be your go-to pieces during this period. While maternity clothes may not yet be necessary, it's never too early to start thinking about building a wardrobe that will evolve with your pregnancy.

Second Trimester: The Bump Appears

The second trimester, often considered the "honeymoon" phase of pregnancy, spans from week 13 to week 26. During this time, many women find that the discomforts of the first trimester, such as morning sickness and fatigue, begin to fade. In their place comes a growing baby bump and other noticeable changes.

Around the middle of the second trimester, your uterus will begin expanding beyond your pelvis, causing your belly to visibly grow. For many women, this is the point where maternity clothes become essential. Your pre-pregnancy pants and skirts may start to feel tight around the waist, and fitted tops may no longer accommodate your expanding midsection. In addition to changes in your belly, you may continue to experience growth in your bust, and your hips may begin to widen in preparation for childbirth.

Dressing for the Second Trimester

The second trimester is when most women start investing in maternity-specific clothing. Look for pieces that provide both comfort and support, such as maternity jeans with stretchy panels, wrap dresses, and tops with ruching or empire waists that flatter your growing belly. This is also the time to invest in supportive bras that accommodate your changing bust size. Maternity leggings, loose skirts, and tunics are great options for maintaining comfort without sacrificing style.

During this stage, you'll want to prioritize clothes that offer flexibility and room to grow, as your body will continue to change rapidly. Additionally, breathable fabrics like cotton and bamboo can help keep you cool, as many women experience fluctuations in body temperature during pregnancy.

Third Trimester: Preparing for Baby

The third trimester, from week 27 to the end of your pregnancy, is when your body reaches its largest and most physically demanding stage. During this time, your baby is rapidly growing, and your belly will expand significantly. Your skin may stretch, and you may experience swelling in your feet, ankles, and hands due to increased fluid retention. Back pain, pressure on your bladder, and difficulty moving comfortably are common issues in the third trimester.

At this stage, comfort is more important than ever. Clothes that were once comfortable may now feel too tight, and you may need to size up or look for maternity-specific pieces that provide ample support. Footwear is also crucial during this time, as swelling in the feet can make tight or high-heeled shoes uncomfortable. Opt for shoes that offer good arch support and are easy to slip on, as bending over to tie laces may become more difficult.

Dressing for the Third Trimester

In the third trimester, you'll likely want to prioritize comfort over everything else. Loose-fitting dresses, maternity pants with over-the-belly support, and tops that don't cling to your belly are ideal. Maxi dresses and stretchy tunics are great for accommodating your growing bump while providing enough flexibility for movement.

Compression socks or leggings can help with swelling, and choosing shoes that are supportive and easy to wear will make a big difference in your daily comfort. At this stage, layering can also be helpful, as it allows you to adjust your clothing as your body temperature fluctuates.

Common Maternity Wardrobe Pitfalls to Avoid

As you build your maternity wardrobe, it's important to be mindful of certain common pitfalls that can make dressing during pregnancy more challenging. Avoiding these mistakes will help you create a wardrobe that is functional, comfortable, and stylish throughout all three trimesters.

1. Buying Too Many Pieces Too Early

One of the most common mistakes pregnant women make is rushing to buy an entirely new maternity wardrobe too early in their pregnancy. While it's natural to feel excited about the changes to come, buying clothes before your body has fully changed can lead to purchasing items that don't fit properly later on. Instead, focus on building your wardrobe gradually as your body changes, ensuring that each piece you buy serves a purpose at that stage.

2. Overlooking Versatility

When shopping for maternity clothes, it's easy to get caught up in buying trendy or overly specific pieces that may not be versatile enough to wear throughout your pregnancy. Instead, focus on items that can be worn multiple ways and dressed up or down. A versatile maternity dress, for example, can be paired with a blazer for work or dressed down with sneakers for a casual outing.

3. Buying Clothes That Are Too Big

Some women assume that buying regular clothes in a larger size will serve as an effective maternity wardrobe. However, this approach often leads to ill-fitting clothing that doesn't flatter your changing shape. Maternity clothes are designed to accommodate your growing bump while still offering structure and support where you need it. Investing in well-fitting maternity clothes, rather than just sizing up, will help you feel more comfortable and confident.

4. Ignoring Fabric Choices

During pregnancy, your skin may become more sensitive, and you may experience fluctuations in body temperature. It's important to choose fabrics that are breathable, soft, and non-restrictive. Natural fibers like cotton, bamboo, and modal are great choices, as they are gentle on the skin and allow for better air circulation. Avoid fabrics that are too stiff, scratchy, or synthetic, as they may cause discomfort.

5. Forgetting About Postpartum Needs

When building your maternity wardrobe, it's essential to consider how your clothes will transition into the postpartum period. Investing in nursing-friendly tops, bras, and dresses will make the transition smoother, allowing you to continue wearing many of your maternity clothes after your baby is born. Look for pieces that are easy to nurse in or that offer enough flexibility for your body's gradual return to its pre-pregnancy shape.

Adapting Your Pre-Pregnancy Wardrobe: What Still Works?

The idea that you need to completely overhaul your wardrobe the moment you become pregnant is a common misconception. In reality, many of your pre-pregnancy clothes can still work for at least part of your pregnancy, especially in the first trimester. By making a few simple adjustments and knowing which pieces to hold onto, you can extend the life of your favorite outfits and create a maternity wardrobe that incorporates items you already own.

1. Stretchy and Flowy Tops

If you have flowy or oversize tops in your pre-pregnancy wardrobe, they can often be worn throughout much of your pregnancy. Loose-fitting blouses, tunics, and stretchy shirts are perfect for accommodating your growing belly without feeling too tight or restrictive. These tops can be paired with maternity leggings or jeans to create comfortable yet stylish outfits for casual or work settings.

2. Leggings and Stretchy Pants

Leggings are a pregnancy staple for many women, and you may find that your pre-pregnancy leggings still fit comfortably during the first and second trimesters. Opt for leggings with a wide, stretchy waistband that sits below your belly. As your pregnancy progresses, you may want to invest in maternity-specific leggings that offer additional support for your growing bump.

3. Empire Waist Dresses

Empire waist dresses are a fantastic option for pregnant women because they feature a high waistline that sits just below the bust, allowing the fabric to flow over your belly without being restrictive. These types of dresses, often already present in many women's wardrobes, are ideal for pregnancy because they provide room for your growing belly while still offering a flattering silhouette. The beauty of empire waist dresses is that they can work through much of your pregnancy, especially in the second and third trimesters, when your bump becomes more pronounced.

You can dress these pieces up or down depending on the occasion, pairing them with sandals or sneakers for casual outings or adding heels or a statement necklace for more formal events.

4. Cardigans and Open Jackets

Another great item you can carry over from your pre-pregnancy wardrobe is cardigans and open jackets. Because these pieces don't need to be buttoned or zipped up over your belly, they can easily accommodate your growing bump while adding style and layers to your outfits. Long cardigans, blazers, and open jackets are perfect for giving structure to a maternity look, especially when worn over stretchy tops or dresses.

These layering pieces are incredibly versatile and can be worn through all stages of pregnancy. During cooler months, you can use them to stay warm without feeling constricted, and they're also great for providing extra coverage or style in professional settings.

5. Maxi Dresses

Maxi dresses are another staple that can easily transition from your pre-pregnancy wardrobe into maternity wear. With their long, flowing design, maxi dresses are not only comfortable but also perfect for accommodating a growing belly. The soft, stretchy fabric used in many maxi dresses makes them ideal for the later stages of pregnancy when comfort is a priority.

These dresses can be worn casually with sandals or accessorized with a belt above your bump to create a more defined shape. Maxi dresses are also wonderful for special occasions like baby showers or maternity photo shoots, as they offer both comfort and elegance.

6. Stretchy Skirts

If you have pre-pregnancy skirts with elastic waistbands or a generous amount of stretch, you may be able to continue wearing them well into your pregnancy. Stretchy skirts, especially those made from soft fabrics like jersey or knit, can sit comfortably below your bump and provide room for movement. These skirts can be paired with maternity or loose-fitting tops for a comfortable yet chic outfit.

If you find that the waistband of the skirt becomes too tight, consider using a belly band, which can help extend the life of your pre-pregnancy skirts and pants by adding a layer of coverage and comfort over your growing belly.

7. Wrap Dresses and Tops

Wrap dresses and tops are incredibly useful during pregnancy because their adjustable design allows you to tighten or loosen them as needed. These pieces can easily adapt to your changing body, making them great for both pregnancy and postpartum wear. Wrap dresses and tops are also nursing-friendly, as they provide easy access for breastfeeding once your baby arrives.

Because they're so versatile, wrap dresses and tops can be worn in both casual and formal settings, depending on how they're styled. Whether you pair them with leggings for a laid-back look or heels for a more polished outfit, they'll give you the flexibility and comfort you need throughout your pregnancy.

Creating a Maternity Capsule Wardrobe

As you adapt your pre-pregnancy wardrobe and invest in maternity pieces, it's helpful to think about building a maternity capsule wardrobe—a collection of essential, versatile pieces that can be mixed and matched to create a variety of outfits. The goal of a capsule wardrobe is to simplify your clothing choices while ensuring that each item serves multiple purposes.

Here are some key pieces to include in your maternity capsule wardrobe:

1. Maternity Jeans with Stretchy Panels

Maternity jeans are an essential part of any pregnancy wardrobe, offering the comfort and support you need as your belly grows. Look for jeans with stretchy panels that either sit under your belly or provide over-the-belly support. These jeans can be dressed up with blouses and jackets or dressed down with t-shirts and cardigans for casual outings.

2. Maternity Leggings

Maternity leggings are one of the most versatile and comfortable items in a maternity wardrobe. Made from stretchy, breathable fabrics, they provide the flexibility and support you need throughout your pregnancy. Pair them with oversize shirts, tunics, or dresses for a comfortable yet stylish look.

3. Wrap Dresses

As mentioned earlier, wrap dresses are a fantastic option for maternity wear. Their adjustable fit makes them suitable for all stages of pregnancy, and they can easily transition into your postpartum wardrobe. Opt for a few wrap dresses in neutral or solid colors that can be accessorized and styled for different occasions.

4. Comfortable, Stretchy Tops

Look for tops made from soft, stretchy fabrics that offer room to grow. Tops with ruching, empire waists, or loose, flowy designs are great options for accommodating your bump. Choose a mix of casual tops for everyday wear and more polished options for work or special occasions.

5. Maternity Bras and Underwear

Your bust will likely grow throughout your pregnancy, so investing in comfortable, supportive maternity bras is essential. Look for bras with adjustable straps and soft, breathable fabrics. You'll also want to choose maternity underwear that provides adequate support and doesn't dig into your skin. Many maternity underwear options offer a high-waisted design that sits comfortably over your bump.

6. Maxi Dresses

As discussed earlier, maxi dresses are a maternity staple that provide comfort, style, and flexibility. Look for a couple of maxi dresses in different colors or patterns to create easy, stylish outfits that can be dressed up or down.

7. Layering Pieces

Layering is key to creating a versatile maternity wardrobe. Cardigans, blazers, and open jackets can be worn over your maternity tops and dresses to create different looks without adding bulk. Choose lightweight layers for warmer months and thicker options for cooler weather.

Conclusion: Building a Wardrobe for Your Changing Body

Understanding your body's changes during pregnancy is the first step in building a maternity wardrobe that supports you through each stage of this trans-formative journey. As your body grows and evolves, your clothing needs will shift, and adapting your wardrobe accordingly will help you stay comfortable and confident.

By investing in versatile, maternity-specific pieces and incorporating items from your pre-pregnancy wardrobe, you can create a collection of clothes that makes dressing easier and more enjoyable. Avoiding common maternity wardrobe pitfalls, such as buying too much too soon or choosing the wrong fabrics, will save you both time and money in the long run.

Ultimately, your maternity wardrobe should reflect both your personal style and the practical needs of your changing body. By prioritizing comfort, versatility, and adaptability, you'll feel empowered to embrace each stage of pregnancy with confidence and grace.

This chapter provides the foundation for understanding how your wardrobe can evolve alongside your pregnancy, setting the stage for deeper discussions on how to dress for different stages, special occasions, and postpartum recovery. Whether you're in your first trimester or preparing for the final weeks before delivery, these wardrobe strategies will help you navigate your pregnancy with style and ease.

Building a Versatile Maternity Wardrobe

A maternity wardrobe should be more than just functional—it should help you feel stylish and confident as your body changes. The key to achieving this balance is building a versatile maternity wardrobe that adapts to different stages of pregnancy, is appropriate for various occasions, and accommodates the changing seasons. By focusing on essential pieces, layering, and smart styling, you can create a collection of clothes that serve you throughout your pregnancy and beyond.

In this chapter, we will explore the essential items every pregnant woman should have for each season, how to mix and match maternity clothing for different occasions, and the must-have maternity pieces that will keep you comfortable and stylish from jeans to Lounge-wear. By the end of this chapter, you'll have a clear strategy for building a wardrobe that supports both your comfort and personal style through all nine months.

Maternity Wardrobe Essentials for Every Season

Pregnancy spans roughly nine months, meaning you'll likely experience at least one, if not multiple, seasons during your journey. Just like in your pre-pregnancy life, dressing for the season is key to staying comfortable. However, as your body changes, your seasonal wardrobe may need to be adjusted to accommodate these new demands. Here's a breakdown of the essential maternity wardrobe pieces you'll need for each season:

1. Spring Maternity Essentials

Spring is often a time of fluctuating weather, with warm days followed by cooler nights. Dressing for this season is all about layering and versatility. You'll want to choose items that can be easily added or removed as the weather changes throughout the day.

- Maternity Jeans or Jeggings: These are essential for spring as they provide comfort and stretch while keeping you warm. Opt for pairs with over-the-belly support or a low-rise waistband that sits comfortably beneath your bump.

- Lightweight Dresses: A lightweight maternity dress, such as a wrap dress or an empire waist design, can be worn on warmer days and layered with a cardigan for cooler mornings and evenings. Choose breathable fabrics like cotton or linen.

- Cardigans or Open Sweaters: A soft cardigan or lightweight sweater is perfect for layering over maternity tops or dresses during the spring. These pieces are great because they don't need to close over your belly, giving you room to grow while still keeping you warm.

- Comfortable Sneakers or Ballet Flats: Spring often means more time spent outdoors, so opt for shoes that provide support and comfort. Ballet flats or slip-on sneakers can be stylish while also accommodating any swelling in your feet.

2. Summer Maternity Essentials

Summer pregnancies can be especially challenging due to the heat and humidity. Lightweight, breathable fabrics and comfortable, loose-fitting clothing are key to staying cool and comfortable during these months.

- Maternity Tank Tops: Soft, stretchy tank tops are a summer must-have. They allow for easy layering and provide breathable coverage for your growing belly. Look for tanks with built-in bras for extra support.

- Maxi Dresses: These long, flowing dresses are ideal for keeping cool in the summer heat. Opt for maxi dresses made from light, breathable fabrics like cotton or bamboo. The loose fit will keep you comfortable while still flattering your figure.

- Maternity Shorts: For particularly hot days, maternity shorts are a lifesaver. Choose styles with elastic waistbands or over-the-belly support for maximum comfort. Pair them with casual tees or tanks for a relaxed look.

- Flip Flops or Sandals: Pregnancy can cause your feet to swell, especially in the heat, so it's essential to choose comfortable footwear. Look for sandals or flip-flops with cushioned soles and adjustable straps to accommodate swelling.

3. Fall Maternity Essentials

Fall is the perfect season for layering. As the weather cools, you'll want to focus on pieces that can transition seamlessly from warm afternoons to chilly evenings.

- Maternity Sweaters: Soft, stretchy maternity sweaters are perfect for fall. Look for styles that provide plenty of room for your bump while still flattering your figure. Long sweaters can be paired with maternity leggings or jeans for a comfortable, stylish look.

- Maternity Scarves: A cozy scarf adds warmth and style to your fall outfits. Plus, it's a great way to add a pop of color or pattern to an otherwise neutral outfit. Opt for lightweight scarves early in the season and switch to heavier options as the weather gets colder.

- Boots: Ankle boots or tall boots are fall staples and can be paired with everything from maternity jeans to dresses. Choose styles with low heels or flat soles for comfort and stability, as your balance may shift as your belly grows.

- Maternity Leggings: Soft, stretchy maternity leggings are perfect for layering under tunics, sweaters, or dresses. Look for leggings with a high waistband that can either sit over or under your belly, depending on your comfort level.

4. Winter Maternity Essentials

Dressing for a winter pregnancy can be challenging, especially if you live in a particularly cold climate. Layering is key, and you'll want to invest in pieces that keep you warm without feeling restrictive.

- Maternity Coats: As your belly grows, your pre-pregnancy coats may no longer fit comfortably. Look for a maternity coat with an adjustable fit or extra room around the belly. Some brands offer coats with zip-in panels that can be expanded as your pregnancy progresses.

- Thermal Tops and Leggings: Thermal tops and leggings are perfect for layering under your regular maternity clothes to keep you warm during the winter months. Choose pieces that are soft and stretchy, so they don't feel restrictive as your bump grows.

- Knit Dresses: A knit maternity dress paired with tights and boots is a stylish and comfortable option for winter. Choose dresses made from warm fabrics like wool or cashmere blends for added warmth.

- Waterproof Boots: Snow or rain can be tricky to navigate during pregnancy, so it's important to have a pair of waterproof boots that offer both warmth and traction. Look for boots with good arch support to keep your feet comfortable as they may swell.

Mixing and Matching for Different Occasions

Building a versatile maternity wardrobe isn't just about buying essentials for each season—it's also about choosing pieces that can be mixed and matched for different occasions. Whether you're dressing for work, a casual weekend, or a special event, having a few key items that can be styled in multiple ways will make getting dressed easier and more enjoyable.

1. Work and Office Wear

If you're working during your pregnancy, you'll want to invest in maternity pieces that are both professional and comfortable. Many maternity brands offer work-friendly options that can easily transition from the office to after-hours events.

- Maternity Blazers: A structured maternity blazer can instantly elevate any outfit. Pair it with maternity trousers or a pencil skirt for a polished office look. For more casual work environments, wear it over a maternity dress or jeans.

- Maternity Trousers: Look for maternity trousers with an elastic waistband or over-the-belly support. Black or navy trousers are versatile enough to be paired with different blouses or tops throughout the week.

- Maternity Dresses: A classic wrap dress or shift dress is a great option for the office. Choose styles that are comfortable but also professional enough for meetings and presentations. You can dress these up with a blazer and heels or down with flats.

2. Casual and Everyday Wear

For casual weekends or days spent running errands, you'll want comfortable maternity clothes that are easy to move in but still stylish enough for stepping out.

- Maternity T-Shirts: Basic maternity t-shirts in neutral colors are wardrobe staples. Pair them with maternity jeans or leggings for a casual, comfortable look. Layer with cardigans or jackets for added style.

- Maternity Jeans: A good pair of maternity jeans can take you through the entire pregnancy. Look for stretchy, supportive styles that can be dressed up or down depending on your plans. Dark-wash jeans can be paired with a blouse and boots for a more polished look, while lighter washes are perfect for casual outings.

- Maternity Hoodies or Sweatshirts: For cozy weekends at home or casual outings, a maternity hoodie or sweatshirt is a must-have. Look for styles that provide plenty of room for your belly while keeping you warm and comfortable.

3. Special Occasions

Whether it's a wedding, baby shower, or holiday event, dressing for special occasions during pregnancy can feel daunting. However, with a few versatile pieces, you can look and feel your best.

- Maternity Cocktail Dresses: Look for maternity dresses that have a flattering fit, such as wrap styles, empire waistlines, or dresses with ruching. These styles will highlight your growing bump while still allowing you to feel comfortable and elegant. Choose fabrics like silk, chiffon, or lace for a more formal look.

- Maternity Jumpsuits: A maternity jumpsuit is a trendy and comfortable option for special occasions. Opt for a black or jewel-toned jumpsuit that can be dressed up with statement jewelry and heels. Jumpsuits offer the perfect balance of comfort and style, making them ideal for weddings or evening events.

- Maternity Skirts: For a more versatile option, maternity skirts can be paired with different tops to create various looks. A black maternity skirt, for example, can be worn with a sequined top for a formal event or with a blouse for a more casual occasion.

Must-Have Maternity Pieces (From Jeans to Lounge-wear)

Now that we've explored how to dress for different seasons and occasions, let's focus on the must-have maternity pieces that will anchor your wardrobe. These items will provide the foundation for a stylish, comfortable, and versatile maternity wardrobe that you can rely on throughout your pregnancy and even beyond. Investing in these key pieces will ensure that you have outfits that work for a variety of settings, whether you're at home, running errands, attending an event, or going to work.

1. Maternity Jeans

Maternity jeans are an absolute must-have for any pregnant woman. They offer the structure and versatility of regular jeans while providing the stretch and comfort necessary to accommodate a growing bump. Maternity jeans come in a variety of styles, including skinny, straight-leg, and boot cut, allowing you to choose the fit that flatters your body and matches your style.

Key Features to Look For:

- Over-the-Belly Support: Some maternity jeans come with a stretchy panel that extends over your belly, providing support and keeping the jeans in place as your bump grows. This style is great for extra support and a seamless look under longer tops.

- Under-the-Belly Waistband: Other maternity jeans have an elastic waistband that sits under your belly, which can be more comfortable for some women, especially in the early stages of pregnancy.

- Stretchy Fabric: Look for jeans made with a blend of cotton, polyester, and spandex for maximum comfort. The fabric should stretch without losing its shape, allowing for a comfortable fit throughout your pregnancy.

Styling Tips:

Maternity jeans are incredibly versatile and can be dressed up or down depending on the occasion. Pair them with a casual t-shirt and sneakers for a relaxed day out, or dress them up with a blouse and a blazer for a more polished look. Dark-wash jeans tend to look more formal, while lighter washes are perfect for casual outings.

2. Maternity Leggings

Few items are as comfortable during pregnancy as a pair of maternity leggings. Made from soft, stretchy fabrics, these leggings can be worn for lounging around the house, running errands, or even dressing up for a casual outing. Maternity leggings are designed to accommodate your growing belly while providing support and flexibility.

Key Features to Look For:

- Over-the-Belly Fit: Many maternity leggings have a high, stretchy waistband that covers your belly, offering support and comfort as your bump expands. This style is especially helpful in later stages of pregnancy when extra belly support is needed.

- Supportive Fabric: Choose leggings made from high-quality, stretchy fabric that provides gentle compression to support your legs and lower back. Fabrics like cotton or modal blended with spandex are ideal for both comfort and durability.

- Seamless Design: Look for leggings with a smooth, seamless design that prevents irritation and offers a sleek silhouette. This is particularly important if you plan to wear them under fitted tops or dresses.

Styling Tips:

Maternity leggings can be paired with long tunics, oversize sweaters, or even maternity dresses for a chic yet comfortable look. For a casual day out, wear them with sneakers and a t-shirt. For a more elevated look, opt for a pair of black leggings, a fitted blouse, and ankle boots.

3. Maternity Dresses

Maternity dresses are a staple in any pregnant woman's wardrobe, offering comfort, ease, and style in one piece. The best maternity dresses are designed to accommodate your growing belly while still flattering your figure. Whether you're attending a formal event or looking for something casual, a good maternity dress can be dressed up or down.

Key Features to Look For:

- Empire Waist or Wrap Styles: Dresses with an empire waist or wrap design are ideal for pregnancy because they highlight the bust while allowing the fabric to flow over your belly, creating a flattering silhouette.

- Stretchy or Flowing Fabric: Opt for dresses made from fabrics like jersey, cotton, or chiffon, which provide stretch and drape nicely over your bump.

- Versatility: Choose dresses that can be worn in multiple settings, such as a maxi dress for summer days, a body con dress for special occasions, or a flowy midi dress for casual outings.

Styling Tips:

Maternity dresses are incredibly easy to style. For a more formal event, choose a fitted dress with ruching around the belly and pair it with heels and statement jewelry. For a casual look, wear a flowy dress with flats or sandals, and accessorize with a lightweight scarf. You can also layer maternity dresses with cardigans, denim jackets, or blazers to suit different occasions.

4. Maternity T-Shirts and Tops

Maternity tops are designed to provide room for your growing belly while still maintaining a flattering fit. These tops come in a variety of styles, including basic t-shirts, blouses, and tunics. A few well-chosen maternity tops will make it easy to mix and match your outfits throughout your pregnancy.

Key Features to Look For:

- Ruching or Draping: Many maternity tops feature ruching along the sides or a draped design that allows the fabric to stretch and grow with your belly. This not only provides extra comfort but also gives the top a flattering shape.

- Soft, Stretchy Fabrics: Look for tops made from soft, breathable fabrics like cotton or modal. These fabrics will keep you comfortable while still providing enough stretch to accommodate your bump.

- Nursing-Friendly Options: If you're planning to breastfeed, consider investing in maternity tops that double as nursing tops. These tops have hidden openings or wrap designs that make breastfeeding more convenient after your baby arrives.

Styling Tips:

Maternity t-shirts and tops are easy to style for casual or professional settings. Pair a basic maternity t-shirt with jeans and sneakers for a laid-back weekend look, or tuck a more structured blouse into maternity trousers for a polished office outfit. Don't forget to accessorize with jewelry or scarves to add personality to your outfit.

5. Maternity Bras and Underwear

As your body changes during pregnancy, you'll need to update your undergarments to ensure proper support and comfort. Maternity bras and underwear are specially designed to accommodate your growing bust and belly while providing the support you need.

Key Features to Look For:
   - Adjustable Straps and Bands: Maternity bras often have adjustable straps and bands to accommodate your changing bust size. Some styles also feature multiple hook-and-eye closures for a customization fit.
   - Soft, Breathable Fabrics: Choose bras and underwear made from soft, breathable fabrics like cotton, which will prevent irritation and keep you comfortable throughout the day.
   - Wire-Free Support: Many women find that wire-free bras provide the best combination of comfort and support during pregnancy. Look for bras with wide, supportive straps and a thick band for added lift.

Styling Tips:
   Invest in both everyday bras and sleep bras for comfort during the day and night. Nursing bras, which feature drop-down cups for easy breastfeeding, are also worth considering if you plan to breastfeed after delivery. As for underwear, look for maternity briefs with a high waistband that sits comfortably over your bump.

6. Lounge-wear and Sleepwear

Comfortable Lounge-wear and sleepwear are essential for relaxing at home and getting a good night's sleep. During pregnancy, your sleep patterns may change, and your pre-pregnancy sleepwear may no longer fit comfortably over your bump.

Key Features to Look For:
  - Loose, Stretchy Fabrics: Look for Lounge-wear and sleepwear made from soft, stretchy fabrics like modal, bamboo, or jersey. These materials provide breath-ability and won't feel restrictive as your body changes.
  - Adjustable Waistbands: Many maternity pajama bottoms and Lounge-wear pieces feature adjustable waistbands that allow you to customize the fit as your belly grows.
  - Nursing-Friendly Designs: If you plan to breastfeed, consider purchasing nursing pajamas that feature easy access for nighttime feedings.

Styling Tips:
  For lounging around the house, pair a loose-fitting maternity top with leggings or joggers. When it comes to sleepwear, opt for a soft, stretchy nightgown or a two-piece pajama set that provides ample room for your growing bump. A comfortable robe is also a great addition to your maternity Lounge-wear, especially for those early postpartum days.

Building a versatile maternity wardrobe is all about choosing pieces that are comfortable, stylish, and adaptable to different stages of pregnancy and various occasions. By investing in maternity essentials—such as jeans, leggings, dresses, tops, bras, and Lounge-wear—you can create a wardrobe that meets your needs while allowing you to express your personal style.

The key to a successful maternity wardrobe is versatility. By selecting items that can be mixed and matched, layered, and worn across different settings, you'll maximize your options without overloading your closet. Whether you're preparing for a day at the office, a casual weekend, or a special event, your maternity wardrobe should help you feel confident and comfortable throughout your pregnancy journey.

With the right pieces in your wardrobe, you'll be able to enjoy this special time in your life, knowing that your clothes are working with your body rather than against it. By focusing on essential items and understanding how to style them for different seasons and occasions, you'll create a maternity wardrobe that not only supports your growing bump but also enhances your overall sense of well-being and style.

Fabrics and Materials That Prioritize Comfort

During pregnancy, comfort is paramount, and what you wear plays a critical role in how you feel as your body undergoes profound changes. One of the most essential factors that contribute to your comfort is the fabric of your clothing. The right fabrics can make a world of difference in keeping you cool, flexible, and feeling good throughout your pregnancy. Choosing fabrics that offer breath-ability, stretch, and softness is key to creating a wardrobe that not only supports your body but also ensures that you look and feel great.

In this chapter, we will explore how to choose the right fabrics for maternity wear, focusing on essential characteristics like breath-ability, stretch, and softness. We'll also dive into sustainable and eco-friendly maternity fashion options, which are becoming increasingly popular among mothers-to-be who want to make conscious choices for both their own health and the environment. By the end of this chapter, you'll have a thorough understanding of the types of fabrics and materials that will provide the best support and comfort throughout your pregnancy.

Choosing the Right Fabrics for Maternity Wear

Pregnancy brings a range of physical changes that can affect your skin, temperature regulation, and overall comfort. Choosing the right fabrics is one of the most important considerations when building your maternity wardrobe. The fabric of your clothing directly impacts how your body feels throughout the day, and wearing the wrong materials can lead to discomfort, irritation, or even overheating.

When selecting fabrics for your maternity clothes, prioritize those that are gentle on your skin, breathable, and have the necessary stretch to accommodate your growing bump. Here are some key considerations for choosing the right fabrics:

1. Natural vs. Synthetic Fabrics

One of the first things to consider when selecting maternity wear is the choice between natural and synthetic fabrics. Each type of fabric has its benefits, but natural fabrics tend to be more breathable and gentle on the skin, making them an excellent choice for pregnancy.

- Natural Fabrics: Natural fabrics, such as cotton, linen, and bamboo, are ideal for maternity wear because they are breathable, hypoallergenic, and soft. These fabrics allow air to circulate around your body, which helps prevent overheating, a common issue during pregnancy. They are also less likely to irritate sensitive skin, which is particularly important as pregnancy can make your skin more prone to irritation and dryness.

- Synthetic Fabrics: Synthetic fabrics, such as polyester and nylon, can be durable and affordable, but they may not provide the same level of comfort as natural fabrics. While some synthetic fabrics have been designed with moisture-wicking properties, others can trap heat and cause you to feel sweaty or uncomfortable. However, many modern maternity clothes use blended fabrics (a mix of natural and synthetic fibers) to offer the best of both worlds—stretch and durability from synthetic fibers combined with the softness and breath-ability of natural fibers.

Best Natural Fabrics for Maternity Wear:
  - Cotton: A popular choice for maternity clothing, cotton is soft, breathable, and hypoallergenic, making it perfect for women with sensitive skin. It's lightweight and allows air to circulate, keeping you cool and comfortable throughout the day.

- Linen: Linen is another natural fabric that works well for maternity wear, especially in hot weather. Its lightweight, breathable nature helps wick moisture away from your skin, keeping you cool and comfortable. While linen can wrinkle easily, its airy texture makes it a great choice for casual maternity dresses and tops.

- Bamboo: Bamboo fabric is gaining popularity in the maternity fashion world due to its incredibly soft texture and sustainability. Bamboo is naturally moisture-wicking and temperature-regulating, making it an ideal choice for women who experience frequent temperature fluctuations during pregnancy. It's also antimicrobial, hypoallergenic, and biodegradable, making it a sustainable option.

Blended Fabrics for Maternity Wear:
  - Modal: Modal is a semi-synthetic fabric made from beech tree pulp. It is incredibly soft and stretchy, making it a popular choice for maternity wear, particularly for items like leggings, Lounge-wear, and underwear. Modal is breathable and has excellent moisture-wicking properties, which helps keep you dry and comfortable throughout the day.

- Jersey Knit: Jersey knit is often made from a blend of cotton and synthetic fibers, offering a lightweight, stretchy, and breathable fabric that's perfect for maternity wear. It drapes well over your body and offers plenty of flexibility, making it ideal for maternity tops, dresses, and sleepwear.

Breath-ability, Stretch, and Softness: What to Look For

Comfort during pregnancy is influenced by several factors, including the breath-ability, stretch, and softness of the fabrics you wear. These three qualities are essential to ensuring that your clothes not only fit well but also feel good against your skin.

1. Breath-ability

As your body works to support both you and your growing baby, you may find yourself feeling warmer than usual, especially as your pregnancy progresses. Breath-ability is one of the most important factors to consider when selecting maternity fabrics, as it helps regulate your body temperature and keeps you cool.

- What is Breath-ability?
    Breath-ability refers to a fabric's ability to allow air to pass through it. Fabrics that are breathable enable heat and moisture to escape from your body, preventing you from overheating. This is particularly important during pregnancy when hormonal changes and an increased metabolic rate can cause your body to produce more heat than usual.

- Best Breathable Fabrics:
    - Cotton: Cotton is a highly breathable fabric that allows air to circulate freely, helping to regulate your body temperature.
    - Linen: Linen is another excellent choice for breath-ability, especially in hot and humid climates.
    - Bamboo: Bamboo fabric is naturally moisture-wicking and breathable, helping to keep you dry and cool.

When choosing maternity clothes, prioritize items made from these fabrics to stay comfortable in warm weather or during physical activity.

2. Stretch

One of the key challenges of dressing during pregnancy is accommodating your growing belly while ensuring that your clothes still fit well and provide freedom of movement. Stretchy fabrics are essential for maternity wear, as they allow your clothes to expand with your body without feeling restrictive.

- What is Stretch?

Stretch refers to a fabric's ability to expand and return to its original shape. Fabrics with good stretch will move with your body, providing comfort and flexibility as your bump grows. Stretchy fabrics are especially important in items like maternity leggings, tops, and dresses, as they help accommodate your changing shape without compromising on fit.

- Best Stretchy Fabrics:
  - Spandex/Elastane: Spandex (also known as elastane) is a synthetic fiber that is often blended with other materials to provide stretch. It allows fabrics to expand and contract, making it a popular choice for maternity leggings, active-wear, and body con dresses.
  - Modal: Modal is a semi-synthetic fabric known for its stretch and softness, making it perfect for maternity underwear and Lounge-wear.
  - Jersey Knit: Jersey knit fabrics, which often contain a blend of cotton and spandex, offer excellent stretch and flexibility, making them ideal for maternity tops and dresses.

When shopping for maternity clothes, look for fabrics with a blend of spandex or elastane to ensure that they can stretch comfortably with your growing belly.

3. Softness

During pregnancy, your skin may become more sensitive due to hormonal changes. Soft fabrics are essential to prevent irritation and ensure that your clothes feel gentle against your skin.

- What is Softness?

Softness refers to how a fabric feels against your skin. Fabrics that are smooth, lightweight, and gentle are less likely to cause irritation, making them ideal for maternity wear. Since pregnancy can make your skin more prone to dryness and sensitivity, it's important to choose soft fabrics that won't rub or chafe.

- Best Soft Fabrics:
  - Modal: Modal is prized for its luxurious softness, making it a great choice for items that come into direct contact with your skin, such as underwear, bras, and Lounge-wear.
  - Cotton: Cotton is naturally soft and breathable, making it a good choice for maternity t-shirts, tops, and sleepwear.
  - Bamboo: Bamboo fabric is incredibly soft, with a smooth texture that feels gentle against sensitive skin.

When selecting maternity clothes, prioritize fabrics that feel soft and comfortable to wear, especially for items that will be worn close to your skin, like bras, underwear, and sleepwear.

Sustainable and Eco-Friendly Maternity Fashion Options

As awareness of environmental issues grows, many women are seeking sustainable and eco-friendly fashion options during pregnancy. Sustainable maternity fashion prioritizes fabrics and materials that have a lower environmental impact, as well as production methods that are ethical and environmentally conscious. Choosing sustainable options not only helps protect the planet but also supports your health by reducing exposure to harmful chemicals and pollutants.

1. The Importance of Sustainability in Maternity Fashion

Maternity fashion is unique in that it's often worn for a relatively short period of time, usually around nine months. As a result, many women find themselves with a wardrobe full of maternity clothes that they no longer need after giving birth. This short life-cycle can contribute to fashion waste, especially if those clothes are made from synthetic materials that don't break down easily in landfills.

By choosing sustainable and eco-friendly maternity wear, you can minimize your environmental impact while still enjoying stylish and comfortable clothing. Sustainable fashion focuses on using renewable resources, reducing waste, and ensuring fair labor practices, making it a conscious choice for expectant mothers who want to make a positive impact on the planet.

2. Sustainable Fabrics for Maternity Wear

When shopping for sustainable maternity wear, look for fabrics that are made from renewable resources and have a lower environmental impact. These fabrics are often produced using environmentally friendly processes, require fewer resources, and are biodegradable. Here are some of the most popular sustainable fabrics for maternity fashion:

- Organic Cotton: Regular cotton production can be water- and pesticide-intensive, but organic cotton is grown without the use of harmful chemicals, making it a more eco-friendly choice. Organic cotton is just as soft, breathable, and comfortable as conventional cotton, but it's better for the environment and for farmers. It's an ideal fabric for maternity basics like t-shirts, leggings, and underwear.

- Bamboo: Bamboo is a highly sustainable resource because it grows quickly without the need for pesticides or fertilizers. Bamboo fabric is incredibly soft, breathable, and naturally moisture-wicking, making it an excellent choice for maternity clothing. Additionally, bamboo is biodegradable, making it an eco-friendly option that doesn't contribute to long-term environmental harm.

- Tencel (Lyocell): Tencel is a fabric made from sustainably sourced wood pulp, usually from eucalyptus, beech, or spruce trees. The production process for Tencel uses a closed-loop system, meaning that water and solvents are recycled, reducing waste. Tencel is soft, breathable, and naturally antimicrobial, making it a great fabric for maternity clothing that's worn close to the skin, such as dresses, leggings, and tops.

- Hemp: Hemp is another eco-friendly fabric that has gained popularity in sustainable fashion. It requires minimal water and no pesticides to grow, making it a low-impact crop. Hemp fabric is durable, breathable, and naturally UV-resistant. While hemp tends to be more structured, it is often blended with other fibers like cotton to create softer maternity garments like dresses and tops.

- Recycled Fabrics: Some maternity brands are using recycled materials to create eco-friendly clothing. For example, recycled polyester is made from post-consumer plastic bottles, which helps reduce plastic waste. Recycled fabrics can offer the same stretch and durability as their conventional counterparts while reducing the environmental impact of producing virgin materials.

3. Choosing Ethical and Sustainable Maternity Brands

Beyond the fabrics themselves, the sustainability of your maternity wardrobe also depends on how the clothes are produced. Ethical and sustainable maternity brands focus not only on using eco-friendly materials but also on ensuring fair labor practices, reducing carbon footprints, and minimizing waste in production.

Here are some factors to consider when choosing sustainable maternity brands:

- Fair Labor Practices: Look for brands that are transparent about their production processes and prioritize fair labor practices. Ethical maternity brands ensure that their workers are paid fair wages and work in safe, healthy conditions.

- Sustainable Packaging: Sustainable brands often go beyond clothing and use eco-friendly packaging materials, such as recycled or biodegradable packaging, to minimize waste.

- Waste Reduction: Many sustainable maternity brands focus on reducing waste by producing smaller, more mindful collections. Some also offer recycling or buy-back programs, allowing you to return your gently used maternity clothes for recycling or resale, reducing fashion waste.

- Local Production: Choosing maternity clothes made by brands that manufacture locally or regionally can help reduce the carbon footprint associated with shipping and transportation.

Popular Sustainable Maternity Brands:
  - Boob Design: A Swedish brand that focuses on sustainable, high-quality maternity and nursing wear made from organic cotton and recycled materials.
  - Hatch: Known for its stylish, high-end maternity clothing, Hatch uses sustainable fabrics like Tencel and organic cotton, and the brand focuses on creating timeless pieces that can be worn beyond pregnancy.
  - Seraphine: A popular maternity brand that has introduced a sustainable collection made from organic cotton, bamboo, and other eco-friendly materials.
  - Kindred Bravely: This brand offers comfortable and eco-conscious

maternity and nursing essentials, often made from sustainable fabrics like bamboo and organic cotton.

The Benefits of Choosing Sustainable Maternity Fashion

Making sustainable fashion choices during pregnancy benefits not only the environment but also your health and well-being. Here are some of the key benefits of opting for sustainable maternity wear:

1. Healthier for You and Your Baby

Choosing eco-friendly fabrics like organic cotton or bamboo means that you're avoiding exposure to harmful chemicals, pesticides, and synthetic dyes that are commonly used in conventional fabric production. This is particularly important during pregnancy, as your skin may be more sensitive, and avoiding unnecessary chemicals helps create a healthier environment for both you and your growing baby.

2. Reducing Your Environmental Impact

Sustainable fabrics and ethical production practices help reduce the environmental impact of clothing production. By choosing eco-friendly maternity wear, you're supporting brands that prioritize water conservation, reduce energy consumption, and minimize the use of toxic chemicals. Sustainable fashion also focuses on reducing waste by creating durable, long-lasting garments, which means fewer clothes end up in landfills.

3. Supporting Ethical Labor Practices

Many sustainable fashion brands are committed to ensuring that their workers are treated fairly and paid a living wage. By choosing maternity wear from ethical brands, you're supporting companies that prioritize the welfare of their workers and promote positive social change within the fashion industry.

4. Investing in Quality, Long-Lasting Pieces

Sustainable fashion tends to focus on quality over quantity. When you invest in eco-friendly maternity clothing, you're likely to find that the garments are well-made, durable, and designed to last throughout your pregnancy and beyond. While sustainable maternity wear may come with a slightly higher price tag, the quality and longevity of the pieces often make them worth the investment.

Tips for Building a Sustainable Maternity Wardrobe

Building a sustainable maternity wardrobe doesn't mean you have to sacrifice style or comfort. Here are some tips for creating a wardrobe that is both eco-friendly and functional:

1. Focus on Versatile, Timeless Pieces

When building your sustainable maternity wardrobe, prioritize versatile pieces that can be mixed and matched for different occasions. For example, a classic maternity dress made from organic cotton or Tencel can be worn to work, on casual outings, or dressed up for special events. Choosing timeless pieces rather than trendy items will ensure that your wardrobe remains stylish and functional even after pregnancy.

2. Choose Quality Over Quantity

Rather than buying a large number of inexpensive maternity clothes, focus on investing in high-quality, sustainable pieces that will last throughout your pregnancy and into the postpartum period. Quality maternity clothes made from durable, eco-friendly fabrics will provide better comfort, fit, and longevity than cheaper alternatives.

3. Consider Secondhand or Maternity Rentals

Since maternity clothes are often worn for only a short period, consider buying secondhand or renting maternity clothes to reduce waste. Many online platforms and local consignment shops offer gently used maternity clothes, allowing you to save money and reduce your environmental impact. Additionally, some maternity rental services allow you to rent stylish, high-end maternity clothes for special occasions or everyday wear, making it easy to dress sustainably without a long-term commitment.

4. Donate or Re-purpose Maternity Clothes After Pregnancy

Once your pregnancy is over, consider donating your maternity clothes to a local charity or selling them through a secondhand marketplace. Many women benefit from gently used maternity clothes, and by donating or reselling your clothes, you're extending the life of those garments and reducing fashion waste. Alternatively, you can re-purpose some maternity clothes for postpartum wear or nursing, especially if they are made from versatile fabrics like bamboo or cotton.

As your body undergoes the trans-formative journey of pregnancy, the fabrics and materials you choose for your maternity wardrobe can greatly enhance your comfort, well-being, and style. By focusing on fabrics that offer breath-ability, stretch, and softness, you can ensure that your clothes move with you, keep you cool, and feel good against your skin. Whether you're dressing for a casual day at home or a special occasion, the right fabrics will provide the support you need throughout your pregnancy.

Furthermore, choosing sustainable and eco-friendly maternity fashion options allows you to make conscious choices that benefit both the environment and your health. By investing in quality pieces made from organic cotton, bamboo, Tencel, and other eco-friendly fabrics, you're supporting ethical practices while also ensuring that your maternity wardrobe is durable, versatile, and stylish.

Building a maternity wardrobe that prioritizes comfort and sustainability is not only good for you and your baby but also for the planet. By making thoughtful choices about the fabrics you wear, you'll enjoy a more comfortable pregnancy and contribute to a healthier, more sustainable fashion industry.

First Trimester Fashion

The first trimester of pregnancy is a time of subtle changes and significant transitions. While you may not be sporting a prominent baby bump just yet, your body is already starting to change in ways that affect how your clothes fit and how comfortable you feel in them. Many women experience bloating, breast tenderness, and fatigue during this phase, making comfort an important priority. At the same time, most women don't start showing until the second trimester, so finding a balance between comfort and style can be challenging during this period.

In this chapter, we'll explore the best style solutions for the first trimester. You'll learn how to dress comfortably while managing the subtle changes in your body, how to invest in key transitional pieces that will grow with you, and tips for hiding your baby bump if you're not ready to share the news with others. By the end of this chapter, you'll have the tools to create a first-trimester wardrobe that prioritizes comfort without sacrificing your personal style.

Styling Your First Trimester: Subtle Changes, Maximum Comfort

In the first trimester, the changes in your body may not be dramatic, but they are enough to impact how you feel in your clothes. Many women experience bloating, slight weight gain, and breast growth, even though their baby bump may not yet be visible. These changes can make it difficult to fit into your pre-pregnancy clothes, but they often don't warrant full maternity wear just yet. The key to first-trimester fashion is to find a balance between accommodating your changing body and maintaining your usual style.

1. Prioritizing Comfort

The first trimester is often accompanied by fatigue, morning sickness, and general discomfort, making it essential to prioritize comfort in your wardrobe. While you may not need maternity clothes just yet, choosing items with soft, stretchy fabrics can help you feel more comfortable throughout the day.

- Elastic Waistbands: One of the most immediate areas where women feel discomfort is around the waist. Bloating and early weight gain can make tight waistbands feel constricting. Instead of opting for full maternity pants, which may be too large at this stage, look for jeans, pants, or skirts with elastic waistbands or adjustable closures. Many women find that leggings and jeggings with stretchy waistbands provide much-needed comfort during this phase.

- Soft, Breathable Fabrics: Your body may feel warmer than usual due to hormonal changes, so it's important to choose breathable, lightweight fabrics like cotton, bamboo, or modal. These materials help regulate your body temperature and prevent overheating, which is especially helpful if you experience hot flashes or general discomfort.

- Loose, Flowing Silhouettes: While your baby bump may not be showing, you might experience bloating, which can make tight-fitting clothes uncomfortable. Loose, flowing silhouettes such as oversize shirts, tunics, and A-line dresses are great options for this stage. These styles provide comfort while still maintaining a polished, stylish look.

2. Adapting Your Existing Wardrobe

One of the best strategies for dressing during the first trimester is to work with what you already have in your wardrobe. Since your body hasn't undergone significant changes yet, many of your pre-pregnancy clothes will still fit with a few minor adjustments. This not only saves money but also allows you to maintain your personal style without the need for an entirely new wardrobe.

- Layering: Layering is a great way to adapt your existing wardrobe to accommodate the subtle changes in your body. A loose, flowy top can be layered under a cardigan or blazer, providing both comfort and style. Layering also allows you to add and remove pieces as your body temperature fluctuates, which is common during pregnancy.

- Using Over-sized or Stretchy Pieces: Many women have oversize or stretchy pieces in their wardrobe that can be worn during the first trimester. Over-sized sweaters, tunics, or stretchy dresses can easily accommodate the early stages of pregnancy without the need for maternity-specific clothing. Pair these items with leggings or comfortable pants to create an outfit that's both stylish and practical.

- Using Belts Strategically: If you're experiencing slight weight gain but don't want to invest in maternity clothes yet, consider using belts to adjust the fit of your outfits. A belt worn above your waist can help define your shape and create a more flattering silhouette, even as your body begins to change.

Investing in Key Transitional Pieces

While many of your pre-pregnancy clothes will still fit during the first trimester, it's worth investing in a few key transitional pieces that will provide comfort and grow with you as your pregnancy progresses. Transitional pieces are versatile items that can be worn throughout the first trimester and well into the second and third trimesters, making them a smart investment for your maternity wardrobe.

1. Leggings and Jeggings

Leggings and jeggings are essential for any pregnancy wardrobe, especially in the first trimester when bloating and early weight gain can make traditional pants feel too tight. These stretchy, form-fitting pieces provide comfort without sacrificing style and can be dressed up or down depending on the occasion.

- Maternity Leggings: While you may not need full maternity leggings in the first trimester, investing in a pair of high-quality, stretchy leggings is a good idea. Look for leggings with a high waistband that sits comfortably above your hips without digging in. As your belly grows, maternity leggings with over-the-belly support will provide extra comfort and support.

- Jeggings: Jeggings offer the look of jeans with the comfort of leggings, making them a great option for casual outfits during the first trimester. Look for jeggings with elastic waistbands or adjustable closures that can grow with you throughout your pregnancy.

2. Wrap Dresses

Wrap dresses are one of the most versatile pieces you can invest in during pregnancy. Their adjustable design allows them to be worn throughout the entire pregnancy, from the first trimester when your bump is small to the third trimester when your belly is more prominent. Wrap dresses also provide a flattering silhouette, highlighting your waist while allowing for comfort and movement.

- Why Wrap Dresses Work: Wrap dresses are designed with an adjustable tie that allows you to customize the fit as your body changes. This makes them ideal for the first trimester when you may be experiencing subtle weight gain or bloating but don't yet need maternity-specific clothes. As your belly grows, you can simply adjust the tie for a comfortable, flattering fit.

- Styling Wrap Dresses: Wrap dresses can be dressed up or down depending on the occasion. For a casual look, pair a wrap dress with sandals or flats and a denim jacket. For a more formal occasion, add heels and statement jewelry. The adjustable fit makes wrap dresses a versatile choice for any event.

3. Maternity Bras

As your breasts grow and become more sensitive during the first trimester, investing in comfortable, supportive bras is essential. Many women experience breast tenderness and swelling early in pregnancy, so finding bras that provide the right support without being too tight or constricting is crucial for maintaining comfort.

- Soft, Wire-Free Bras: Many women find that their pre-pregnancy bras become uncomfortable during the first trimester, especially if they contain underwire. Wire-free bras made from soft, stretchy fabrics are a great alternative. These bras provide support without digging into your skin, making them ideal for sensitive breasts.

- Adjustable or Nursing Bras: As your body continues to change, it's helpful to invest in bras that offer adjustable sizing or can double as nursing bras. Maternity bras with adjustable straps and multiple hook closures allow you to customize the fit as your breasts grow. Nursing bras, which feature drop-down cups for breastfeeding, are also a practical choice if you plan to breastfeed after your baby is born.

4. Loose-Fitting Tops and Tunics

Loose-fitting tops and tunics are ideal for the first trimester because they provide room for movement while still looking stylish. These pieces can be paired with leggings, jeans, or skirts to create comfortable, versatile outfits that can be worn in both casual and professional settings.

- Flowy Fabrics: Look for tops made from lightweight, flowy fabrics like cotton or chiffon. These materials will drape nicely over your body without feeling too tight or restrictive, making them perfect for the early stages of pregnancy.

- Layering with Tunics: Tunics are a great layering piece for the first trimester. They can be worn over leggings or jeggings for a comfortable, casual look, or paired with dress pants for a more professional outfit. Look for tunics with adjustable waistlines or side ruching, which will accommodate your growing belly as your pregnancy progresses.

Style Tips for Hiding Your Baby Bump (If Desired)

While some women are eager to show off their baby bump as soon as it appears, others may prefer to keep their pregnancy under wraps during the first trimester. Whether you're waiting to share the news with friends and family or simply want to keep your changing body private, there are several style tricks you can use to discreetly hide your baby bump in the early stages of pregnancy.

1. Opt for Loose, Flowy Silhouettes

One of the easiest ways to hide your baby bump is to choose clothing with loose, flowy silhouettes. Tops and dresses that drape away from the body can help conceal any early signs of pregnancy, such as slight weight gain or bloating.

- Empire Waistlines: Dresses and tops with an empire waistline, which sit just below the bust and flow outward, are particularly effective at hiding a small baby bump. This style draws attention to your upper body while allowing the fabric to fall loosely over your midsection.

- A-Line Dresses: A-line dresses, which are fitted at the top and gradually flare out toward the bottom, are another great option for hiding a baby bump during the first trimester. The flare of the dress creates a flattering silhouette while leaving room for any early pregnancy changes. A-line dresses are versatile and can be styled for both casual and formal occasions, making them a go-to piece when you want to keep things discreet.

2. Use Layers to Your Advantage

Layering is an effective way to hide a growing bump, especially in the early stages of pregnancy. Strategic layering adds depth to your outfit and draws attention away from your midsection, making it easier to keep your pregnancy under wraps.

- Cardigans and Blazers: Wearing a cardigan, blazer, or lightweight jacket over your outfit can create visual interest and add structure, helping to conceal your belly. These pieces also offer the flexibility of being taken off if you get too warm, which is particularly helpful during pregnancy when body temperature can fluctuate.

- Scarves and Shawls: Scarves and shawls can serve as both accessories and functional pieces for hiding a baby bump. A large, draped scarf around your neck or shoulders can help draw attention upward, away from your midsection. Opt for scarves in lightweight fabrics for warmer months and heavier ones for colder weather.

- Vests and Over-sized Coats: Vests and oversize outerwear are stylish and functional options for layering. These pieces can help mask the changes in your midsection without appearing bulky. Pair them with fitted tops underneath to create a balanced look.

3. Dark Colors and Prints

Dark colors and bold prints are useful tools for creating a visually slimming effect, making them great options for concealing a small bump. Dark colors, such as black, navy, and deep jewel tones, tend to minimize the appearance of any bumps or bulges, while prints can distract the eye and draw attention away from your belly.

- Opt for Patterns: Wearing clothing with patterns or prints can help camouflage subtle changes in your body. Florals, geometric shapes, or abstract prints can be especially effective at diverting attention away from your midsection. Choose patterns that are medium to large in size, as small, intricate patterns can sometimes accentuate curves.

- Monochromatic Outfits: Wearing a monochromatic outfit—where the top and bottom are the same color—creates a seamless line that elongates your figure and detracts from any noticeable changes in your body shape. For example, a navy top paired with matching navy pants or a black dress with black tights can help create a sleek, discreet look.

4. Focus on Your Upper Body

Another way to draw attention away from your belly is by highlighting your upper body. By choosing tops and dresses that emphasize your neckline, shoulders, or bust, you can shift the focus of your outfit to these areas, making it less likely that people will notice any early pregnancy changes.

- Off-the-Shoulder Tops: Off-the-shoulder tops or dresses that expose your collarbones and shoulders can help draw attention upward, away from your belly. This style is flattering and feminine, providing a balance between style and comfort.

- Statement Necklaces or Earrings: Accessories like bold necklaces or statement earrings can help divert attention to your face and upper body. Adding an eye-catching necklace or a pair of large earrings will create a focal point higher up, minimizing focus on your midsection.

- Structured Necklines: Tops and dresses with interesting necklines, such as boat necks, V-necks, or sweetheart necklines, can emphasize your upper body while still providing comfort. These styles are particularly effective for drawing attention to your shoulders and bust, helping to maintain a balanced silhouette.

5. Cinched Styles

While it may seem counterintuitive, some women find that strategically cinching their waist with a belt or choosing clothing with defined waistlines can help conceal early pregnancy changes. This technique works especially well when your bump is still small, as it can create a flattering shape without drawing attention to your belly.

- Empire Waist and Cinched Waistlines: Clothing with an empire waist or cinched waistline, where the fabric gathers just below the bust, creates a structured look that can disguise a growing belly. These styles emphasize the narrowest part of your torso while allowing the fabric to flow over your midsection, making them ideal for early pregnancy.

- Using Belts Strategically: If you're wearing a dress or tunic that lacks structure, consider adding a belt just below your bust. This will create the illusion of a defined waist without drawing attention to your belly. A wide, stretchy belt can be particularly useful for creating this effect.

The first trimester of pregnancy is a time of transition, both physically and emotionally. While your body is undergoing subtle changes, dressing in a way that prioritizes comfort while maintaining your personal style is key to feeling confident and at ease during this phase. By focusing on loose, flowing silhouettes, stretchy fabrics, and layering, you can adapt your wardrobe to accommodate the early stages of pregnancy without sacrificing your sense of style.

Investing in key transitional pieces like leggings, wrap dresses, and comfortable bras will not only make you feel more comfortable but also ensure that your wardrobe can grow with you as your pregnancy progresses. These versatile items will provide support and flexibility throughout the first trimester and beyond.

For those who aren't ready to share the news of their pregnancy, there are plenty of style tricks to discreetly hide your baby bump. Whether you're opting for loose, flowy tops, layering with scarves and jackets, or using dark colors and prints, you can dress in a way that makes you feel comfortable while keeping your pregnancy private.

Ultimately, the goal of first-trimester fashion is to make sure you feel both comfortable and stylish as your body begins to change. By incorporating these strategies into your wardrobe, you'll be able to navigate the early stages of pregnancy with confidence, knowing that your clothes are working with your body rather than against it.

Second Trimester Fashion

The second trimester of pregnancy, often referred to as the "honeymoon" period, is a time when many women begin to experience the most visible changes in their body. This is the phase when your baby bump begins to emerge, and while the first-trimester discomforts like morning sickness may have eased, new challenges arise—particularly when it comes to dressing your growing bump. Fashion during the second trimester should be about finding flattering silhouettes that make you feel comfortable and confident, whether you're at work, enjoying a casual day, or attending a special occasion.

This chapter will guide you through the key elements of second-trimester fashion, focusing on how to dress your growing bump in a way that flatters your changing figure. You'll learn how to adapt your wardrobe for different occasions, from professional settings to weekend outings, and discover comfortable lingerie and underwear options that cater to your shifting body shape.

Dressing the Growing Bump: Flattering Silhouettes

As your belly grows during the second trimester, your body begins to take on new proportions that may be unfamiliar. This is the stage where you may no longer fit into many of your pre-pregnancy clothes, and the need for maternity-specific pieces becomes more apparent. However, dressing the bump doesn't mean sacrificing style—many silhouettes are specifically designed to flatter your new shape, offering comfort while highlighting your baby bump in a beautiful and confident way.

1. Embracing Your New Shape

The second trimester is the ideal time to start embracing your baby bump. Rather than hiding it, this is the phase where you can celebrate it by wearing clothes that show off your growing belly in a flattering way. Finding the right silhouettes will help you look and feel your best as your body undergoes these exciting changes.

- Empire Waist: Dresses and tops with an empire waist are among the most flattering silhouettes for pregnant women. The empire waistline sits just below the bust, allowing the fabric to flow gently over the belly. This style enhances the bust while providing plenty of room for your growing bump, creating a feminine and flattering look. Empire waist dresses are perfect for both casual wear and more formal occasions, making them a versatile choice for your maternity wardrobe.

- Wrap Dresses and Tops: Wrap-style dresses and tops are incredibly flattering during pregnancy because they are adjustable and can be cinched at the narrowest part of your body, just below your bust. The wrap design also allows for easy adjustment as your belly grows, offering flexibility and comfort throughout the second and third trimesters. This silhouette emphasizes your waist while allowing your belly to be the star of the outfit, giving you a chic and polished look.

- A-Line Dresses: A-line dresses flare out gradually from the waist, providing a flattering silhouette that accommodates your growing bump. This style creates a balanced look, making it ideal for women who want to highlight their belly without feeling too restricted. A-line dresses are available in a wide range of fabrics, from lightweight cotton for everyday wear to silk or chiffon for formal events.

- Body-con Dresses: For those who want to accentuate their bump, body con dresses are a popular choice. Made from stretchy, form-fitting fabrics, these dresses hug your curves and proudly showcase your baby bump. Body-con dresses can be casual or dressy, depending on how you style them. Pair a body con dress with a denim jacket and sneakers for a casual look, or dress it up with heels and a statement necklace for a night out.

2. Opting for Stretchy and Adjustable Fabrics

The second trimester is marked by rapid changes in your body size, particularly around your belly and breasts. To accommodate these changes, it's essential to choose fabrics that offer stretch and flexibility, allowing your clothes to grow with you while maintaining their shape.

- Jersey Knit: Jersey knit fabrics are soft, stretchy, and breathable, making them ideal for maternity wear. This fabric drapes beautifully over your bump and provides enough stretch to keep you comfortable as your body grows. Jersey knit is commonly used in maternity tops, dresses, and leggings because of its flexibility and comfort.

- Modal: Modal is another stretchy fabric that is perfect for pregnancy. It's soft, lightweight, and breathable, making it ideal for both casual and dressy maternity pieces. Modal is commonly used in maternity t-shirts, dresses, and sleepwear because of its softness and ability to stretch without losing its shape.

- Ruching and Side Panels: Maternity clothes with ruching along the sides or stretchy side panels are great for the second trimester because they offer extra room for your growing belly. Ruching helps the fabric expand without looking bulky, while side panels allow for flexibility in pants, skirts, and dresses.

Adapting Your Style for Work, Play, and Special Occasions

The second trimester often brings a renewed sense of energy and well-being, making it a great time to enjoy various activities—whether you're heading to work, spending a weekend outdoors, or attending a special occasion. However, as your body changes, your wardrobe may need to adapt to different environments and situations. This section will guide you through creating stylish and comfortable outfits for different occasions, ensuring that you feel confident and fashionable no matter where you are.

1. Dressing for Work: Professional and Polished

Dressing for work during pregnancy can be challenging, especially if your office environment requires professional attire. Fortunately, many maternity brands offer work-appropriate pieces that are both stylish and comfortable, allowing you to maintain a polished look while accommodating your growing bump.

- Maternity Blazers: A tailored maternity blazer is a great investment for your work wardrobe. Look for blazers with a little extra room around the belly or ones that feature side panels or stretch fabric. Pair your blazer with maternity trousers or a pencil skirt for a classic, professional look.

- Maternity Trousers: Maternity trousers with an elastic waistband or over-the-belly support are essential for a professional wardrobe. Black or navy trousers can be easily paired with blouses, sweaters, or blazers to create a variety of polished outfits. Look for trousers made from stretchy, breathable fabrics that allow for movement and comfort throughout the day.

- Shift Dresses: Maternity shift dresses are another great option for work. Their loose, straight silhouette is both flattering and professional, and they can be easily dressed up with a blazer or scarf. Shift dresses in neutral colors like black, gray, or navy are versatile and can be worn multiple times throughout your pregnancy.

2. Dressing for Play: Casual and Comfortable

Whether you're running errands, spending a weekend outdoors, or simply lounging at home, it's important to have casual outfits that are comfortable and easy to wear. The second trimester is a time when you can start experimenting with maternity-specific clothing that offers comfort without sacrificing style.

- Maternity Jeans: Maternity jeans are a must-have for casual wear. Look for jeans with a stretchy waistband or over-the-belly support that grows with you. Skinny or straight-leg maternity jeans can be paired with casual tops, t-shirts, or sweaters for a relaxed look. Dark-wash jeans tend to be more versatile, as they can be dressed up or down depending on the occasion.

- Leggings and Joggers: For ultimate comfort, maternity leggings and joggers are essential. Look for leggings with a high waistband that sits comfortably over your belly, offering both support and flexibility. Joggers made from soft, stretchy fabric are perfect for casual outings or lounging at home. Pair them with a loose-fitting top or hoodie for a cozy, laid-back look.

- Casual Dresses: Maxi dresses, t-shirt dresses, and wrap dresses are all great options for casual wear during the second trimester. These dresses provide comfort and flexibility while still looking stylish. Maxi dresses are especially popular for summer pregnancies, as they are lightweight, breathable, and easy to throw on for a quick outing.

3. Dressing for Special Occasions: Elegant and Comfortable

Whether you're attending a wedding, baby shower, or other formal event, dressing for special occasions during the second trimester can be fun and exciting. With the right maternity pieces, you can look elegant and stylish while still feeling comfortable.

- Maternity Cocktail Dresses: For formal events, maternity cocktail dresses with empire waistlines, ruching, or wrap designs are perfect for showcasing your bump in a flattering way. Look for dresses made from soft, stretchy fabrics like silk, jersey, or chiffon, which provide both comfort and style. Bold colors like jewel tones or classic black are timeless and elegant choices for evening events.

- Maxi Dresses for Special Occasions: Maxi dresses are another versatile option for formal events. Opt for maxi dresses with a fitted bodice and a flowing skirt that drapes over your bump. Floral patterns, lace details, or satin fabrics can elevate a maxi dress for a more formal setting.

- Statement Accessories: To complete your special occasion look, don't forget to add accessories. Statement jewelry, a chic clutch, and a pair of comfortable heels or dressy flats can take your outfit to the next level. Make sure to choose shoes that provide support and comfort, especially as your feet may swell during pregnancy.

Comfortable Underwear and Lingerie for Changing Body Shapes

During pregnancy, your body undergoes significant changes that affect not only your outerwear but also your underwear and lingerie. As your breasts grow and your hips expand, you'll need to invest in underwear and lingerie that provide the right support, comfort, and flexibility for your changing shape.

1. Maternity Bras

One of the most noticeable changes during pregnancy is the growth of your breasts. As they prepare for breastfeeding, your breasts may become larger and more sensitive, making it essential to find bras that offer support without being too restrictive.

- Soft-Cup Bras: Soft-cup bras, which are free of underwire, are a popular choice for pregnant women. These bras provide gentle support without the discomfort of underwire, which can dig into your skin as your breasts grow. Soft-cup bras are often made from stretchy, breathable fabrics like cotton or bamboo, providing flexibility as your bust size changes throughout your pregnancy.

- Maternity and Nursing Bras: Many maternity bras double as nursing bras, offering features like drop-down cups for easy breastfeeding access after your baby is born. These bras are designed to accommodate both the increased size of your breasts during pregnancy and the practical needs of nursing postpartum. Look for bras with adjustable straps, wide bands, and multiple hook-and-eye closures so you can customize the fit as your body changes.

- Supportive Sports Bras: As your breasts grow and become more sensitive, you may want extra support for exercise or everyday activities. A supportive maternity sports bra can help reduce discomfort during physical activity. Look for sports bras with a wide band under the bust and padded straps for added support and comfort.

2. Maternity Underwear

Your changing belly, hips, and pelvic region require underwear that fits comfortably without causing irritation or pressure. Maternity underwear is specifically designed to offer flexibility and support for your changing body, with various styles to choose from.

- Over-the-Belly Panties: These panties provide full coverage, with a waistband that sits over your bump, offering support and comfort. Over-the-belly panties are great for women who prefer more coverage and want their underwear to provide gentle compression over their belly. These styles are particularly comfortable during the later stages of pregnancy when your belly is at its largest.

- Under-the-Belly Panties: For women who prefer a lower-rise style, under-the-belly panties sit comfortably below your bump, offering freedom of movement and a less restrictive feel. These panties are often made from soft, stretchy materials that hug your body without digging into your skin, making them ideal for the second trimester when your belly is growing but not yet at its full size.

- Seamless Panties: Many pregnant women find that seamless panties offer the best combination of comfort and style. These panties are made without irritating seams, making them less likely to cause discomfort or chafing as your body changes. Seamless underwear often comes in both over-the-belly and under-the-belly styles, allowing you to choose the option that best fits your comfort needs.

3. Comfortable Sleepwear and Lounge-wear

Sleep is especially important during pregnancy, but as your body grows, finding comfortable sleepwear that accommodates your changing shape can be challenging. Maternity sleepwear and Lounge-wear are designed to provide extra room and comfort, allowing you to rest more easily.

- Nightgowns and Sleep Shirts: Loose-fitting nightgowns and sleep shirts are ideal for pregnant women who want comfort without restriction. Look for nightgowns made from soft, breathable fabrics like cotton or bamboo, which will keep you cool and comfortable throughout the night. Many maternity nightgowns also double as nursing gowns, with easy-access features like snap buttons or wrap designs.

- Maternity Pajama Sets: Pajama sets with a loose-fitting top and elastic-waist pants are another great option for sleep and lounging. Look for pajama pants with an adjustable waistband or over-the-belly support to accommodate your growing bump. Stretchy, soft fabrics like jersey or modal will provide comfort while ensuring flexibility as your body changes.

- Maternity Robes: A maternity robe is a versatile addition to your Lounge-wear collection. Robes are perfect for layering over your sleepwear, especially during the cooler months, and can also be used postpartum as a comfortable and practical option for nursing.

The second trimester is an exciting time of growth and transformation, and finding the right fashion solutions for your changing body is key to feeling confident and comfortable. From embracing flattering silhouettes like empire waistlines, wrap dresses, and body con styles, to investing in stretchy and supportive fabrics, you can build a wardrobe that highlights your growing bump while keeping you at ease.

Adapting your style for different occasions—whether you're at work, relaxing on the weekend, or attending a special event—ensures that you feel prepared and fashionable no matter the setting. Professional maternity wear like blazers, trousers, and shift dresses can help you maintain a polished look, while casual staples like maternity jeans, leggings, and casual dresses provide comfort for everyday activities. For special occasions, maternity cocktail dresses, maxi dresses, and bold accessories allow you to celebrate your bump in style.

As your body continues to change, finding comfortable and supportive underwear, bras, and sleepwear becomes even more important. Maternity lingerie and underwear are designed to accommodate your growing belly and breasts, providing both comfort and functionality. With the right maternity bras, panties, and sleepwear, you can feel supported and at ease as your pregnancy progresses.

Ultimately, second-trimester fashion is about embracing your new shape, investing in versatile pieces that grow with you, and ensuring that your wardrobe reflects your personal style while meeting the practical needs of your changing body. With these style solutions, you'll feel empowered to enjoy this exciting stage of pregnancy with confidence and grace.

Third Trimester Fashion

The third trimester of pregnancy marks the final stretch before meeting your baby, and it's also the phase where your body undergoes the most dramatic changes. Your belly has expanded significantly, and daily activities may start to feel more physically challenging. Dressing during this stage can be tricky as you balance the need for comfort, support, and style. While your priority may be comfort, there are plenty of ways to dress fashionably in the third trimester, allowing you to maintain your personal style while feeling your best.

In this chapter, we'll explore how to prioritize comfort without sacrificing style, offer tips on finding the perfect maternity dresses and maxi styles, and discuss layering techniques for optimal comfort in any weather. By the end of this chapter, you'll have a thorough understanding of how to dress confidently and comfortably during the final weeks of your pregnancy.

Prioritizing Comfort Without Sacrificing Style

As your body reaches its peak growth during the third trimester, comfort becomes the most critical aspect of your wardrobe. However, just because you're prioritizing comfort doesn't mean you have to give up on style. The key is to find clothes that provide both, ensuring that you feel good and look great as you prepare for the arrival of your baby.

1. Opt for Breathable, Stretchy Fabrics

The third trimester is often accompanied by increased body temperature and swelling, so choosing breathable fabrics is essential. Natural fabrics like cotton, bamboo, and modal are great options for staying cool and comfortable while providing the softness you need for sensitive skin. Breathable fabrics also help prevent overheating, which can be especially uncomfortable during pregnancy.

- Cotton: Cotton is a natural, lightweight fabric that allows air to circulate and keeps you cool. It's perfect for casual everyday wear, from t-shirts to tunics and dresses. Cotton is also easy to layer, making it ideal for transitional weather.

- Bamboo: Bamboo is soft, moisture-wicking, and temperature-regulating, making it an excellent choice for maternity wear during the third trimester. Whether you're looking for Lounge-wear, active-wear, or sleepwear, bamboo fabrics provide the comfort and breath-ability you need as your body changes.

- Modal: Modal is a semi-synthetic fabric made from beech tree pulp. It's incredibly soft, smooth, and breathable, making it perfect for maternity dresses, leggings, and sleepwear. Modal's stretchy nature also accommodates your growing belly without feeling restrictive.

2. Choose Adjustable and Maternity-Specific Styles

As your belly grows, your need for flexibility in your wardrobe increases. Clothing designed with maternity-specific features like stretchy panels, ruching, and adjustable waistbands will offer maximum comfort while still fitting your changing shape. Investing in maternity clothes designed for the third trimester ensures that you're supported where you need it most.

- Ruching: Maternity tops and dresses with side ruching are ideal for the third trimester because they provide extra room for your expanding belly. Ruching allows the fabric to stretch without looking bulky, creating a flattering silhouette that hugs your curves in all the right places.

- Over-the-Belly Support: Maternity leggings and pants with over-the-belly support help alleviate some of the pressure on your lower back and pelvis by offering gentle support to your belly. This added support can make daily activities more comfortable as your belly grows larger.

- Wrap and Empire Waist Styles: Wrap dresses and tops are highly adjustable, making them a perfect choice for the third trimester. The adjustable fit allows you to loosen the wrap as your belly expands, providing both comfort and style. Empire waist dresses, which have a waistband that sits just below the bust, are another flattering option for the third trimester. This silhouette emphasizes your upper body while allowing the fabric to flow gracefully over your belly.

3. Prioritize Footwear Comfort

Foot and ankle swelling are common in the third trimester, so choosing comfortable, supportive footwear is essential. Look for shoes with arch support, cushioned insoles, and easy slip-on designs to accommodate swelling and make getting dressed easier.

- Slip-On Shoes: Bending over to tie shoes can become difficult in the third trimester, so slip-on shoes or sandals are a practical choice. Look for shoes with flexible materials and adjustable straps to ensure they fit comfortably even if your feet swell.

- Supportive Sandals: Sandals with cushioned soles and good arch support are ideal for warmer weather. Opt for styles with wide straps or adjustable buckles that can accommodate changes in your foot size.

- Low-Heeled or Flat Boots: If you're dressing for cooler weather, low-heeled or flat boots with plenty of room in the toe box are a great option. These boots offer stability and support, helping to prevent discomfort and balance issues as your body's center of gravity shifts.

Finding the Perfect Maternity Dresses and Maxi Styles

Maternity dresses and maxi styles are among the most popular choices for women in the third trimester because they offer a combination of comfort, style, and flexibility. Whether you're dressing for a casual outing or a more formal event, the right maternity dress can flatter your bump while providing plenty of room for movement.

1. Empire Waist Dresses

Empire waist dresses are one of the most flattering and comfortable options for pregnant women in the third trimester. This style features a high waistline that sits just below the bust, allowing the fabric to flow loosely over the belly. Empire waist dresses highlight the narrowest part of your body, creating a balanced and elegant silhouette while giving your bump room to grow.

- Why Empire Waist Works: Empire waist dresses provide a comfortable fit without feeling restrictive. They draw attention to your upper body and allow the fabric to drape naturally over your belly, making them perfect for both casual and formal occasions. Choose dresses made from soft, stretchy fabrics like cotton or jersey for added comfort.

- Styling Empire Waist Dresses: Pair an empire waist dress with a lightweight cardigan or blazer for a polished look. You can also accessorize with a statement necklace or earrings to draw attention to your upper body. For casual outings, pair your dress with flat sandals or slip-on shoes for maximum comfort.

2. Wrap Dresses

Wrap dresses are another excellent choice for the third trimester because they offer an adjustable fit that can be customized as your belly grows. The wrap style cinches just below the bust, creating a flattering silhouette that emphasizes your waist while allowing plenty of room for your belly. Wrap dresses are versatile enough to be worn for both casual and formal occasions.

- Adjust-ability of Wrap Dresses: The beauty of wrap dresses lies in their adjust-ability. As your body changes, you can loosen the wrap to create more space around your belly. This makes wrap dresses an ideal option for the third trimester, as they can adapt to your changing shape while still looking chic.

- Styling Wrap Dresses: For a casual daytime look, pair your wrap dress with flats or sneakers. If you're attending a special event, dress it up with heels or wedges and add a statement accessory like a bold necklace or clutch.

3. Maxi Dresses

Maxi dresses are a staple of third-trimester fashion because of their flowing, comfortable design and versatility. Maxi dresses are typically long, reaching down to the ankles, and they are often made from lightweight, breathable fabrics that keep you cool while offering plenty of room for your growing belly.

- Why Maxi Dresses Are Ideal: Maxi dresses provide full coverage while still being incredibly comfortable. The loose fit allows for airflow, making them perfect for warmer weather, and their length makes them suitable for both casual and formal occasions. Maxi dresses are available in various styles, from tank tops to halter necklines, giving you plenty of options to suit your personal style.

- Styling Maxi Dresses: For a relaxed daytime look, wear a maxi dress with flat sandals and a wide-brimmed hat. If you're attending a formal event, pair your dress with statement jewelry, a sleek clutch, and heeled sandals or wedges. Maxi dresses also work well with layers like shawls or cropped jackets, which can be added for extra warmth or style.

4. Body-con Dresses

For women who want to proudly showcase their bump, body con dresses made from stretchy, form-fitting fabrics are an excellent option. Body-con dresses hug your curves and highlight your baby bump, creating a sleek, stylish look that's perfect for a night out or special occasion.

- Comfortable Stretch: Body-con dresses are typically made from materials like jersey or spandex, which offer plenty of stretch to accommodate your changing body. Look for dresses with side ruching or stretchy panels that allow for a comfortable fit throughout the third trimester.

- Styling Body-con Dresses: Pair a body con dress with low heels or ankle boots for a chic evening look. You can also layer it with a blazer or long cardigan for added coverage. Accessories like statement earrings or a bold clutch can elevate your outfit for a special event.

Layering Techniques for Optimal Comfort in Any Weather

As your pregnancy progresses, the weather may change, and so might your body's temperature regulation. Layering is an effective way to ensure you stay comfortable, regardless of the climate. Whether you're navigating the heat of summer or the chill of winter, layering techniques allow you to adapt your outfits for maximum comfort and style.

1. Layering for Warm Weather

Even in warm weather, layering can help you stay cool and comfortable while also allowing you to adjust your outfit as needed. Lightweight layers made from breathable fabrics are key to creating a comfortable summer look.

- Light Cardigans and Kimono Jackets: A lightweight cardigan or kimono jacket can be layered over a tank top or sleeveless dress for extra coverage without adding too much warmth. These pieces are easy to take off if you get too hot, and they add a stylish touch to your outfit.

- Loose Scarves and Shawls: Lightweight scarves or shawls can be a great addition to your summer maternity wardrobe. They offer coverage from the sun or an extra layer in air-conditioned environments without making you overheat. Opt for fabrics like cotton, linen, or silk that are breathable and lightweight.

- Breathable Undergarments: When layering in warm weather, it's essential to choose breathable undergarments. Maternity bras and underwear made from moisture-wicking fabrics like bamboo or modal can help keep you cool and comfortable throughout the day. These fabrics allow air to circulate, reducing the risk of overheating and discomfort.

2. Layering for Cool Weather

As the weather cools down, layering becomes even more important for maintaining warmth and comfort, especially during the third trimester when your body may be more sensitive to temperature changes. Choosing the right layers can help you stay cozy without feeling restricted.

- Chunky Cardigans and Sweaters: Chunky, oversize cardigans and sweaters are perfect for layering over maternity tops and dresses. These pieces provide warmth without being too tight around your growing belly. Look for cardigans with an open front that can easily accommodate your expanding bump. You can also choose sweaters with side slits or a looser fit for added comfort.

- Maternity Coats: As your belly grows, your pre-pregnancy coats may no longer fit comfortably. A maternity coat with extra room around the belly or adjustable features like a zip-in panel can provide the warmth you need while accommodating your changing shape. Some maternity coats also come with features like drawstring waists or expandable sides, making them versatile enough to wear throughout your pregnancy and even postpartum.

- Thermal Layers: For extra warmth in cold weather, thermal tops and leggings can be worn as a base layer under your regular clothes. Thermal layers made from materials like merino wool or fleece provide insulation without adding bulk, helping to keep you warm while allowing for movement and flexibility.

- Scarves, Hats, and Gloves: Accessorizing with scarves, hats, and gloves not only adds a stylish touch to your winter maternity outfits but also provides essential warmth. Choose soft, stretchy materials like wool or cashmere that are gentle on sensitive skin and offer plenty of flexibility for layering over your clothes.

3. Versatile Layering Pieces

No matter the season, having a few versatile layering pieces in your maternity wardrobe can help you create a variety of outfits that work for any weather or occasion. These items can be mixed and matched with your existing wardrobe to ensure you stay comfortable while still looking stylish.

- Maternity Cardigans: A maternity cardigan is a versatile piece that can be worn over dresses, tops, or even Lounge-wear. Choose cardigans with a longer length or an open-front design, as these styles are easier to wear over a growing belly. Cardigans made from lightweight materials like cotton or knit blends can be worn year-round.

- Denim Jackets: A classic denim jacket is another great layering piece that works well with casual outfits. Its structured yet casual look pairs nicely with maxi dresses, leggings, or jeans. Since denim jackets typically don't need to close over your belly, they're perfect for adding a bit of edge to your maternity wardrobe while still being comfortable.

- Ponchos and Capes: Ponchos and capes offer stylish and comfortable layering options that work especially well in cooler weather. Their loose, flowy design allows for plenty of movement, and they can be easily thrown over any outfit for extra warmth. Ponchos made from soft, cozy materials like wool or knit blends are perfect for layering over dresses or pants during the third trimester.

4. Layering for Transitional Weather

During transitional seasons like spring and fall, layering becomes especially important as temperatures can fluctuate throughout the day. The goal is to have enough layers to keep you warm in the cooler mornings and evenings while allowing you to adjust as the weather warms up during the day.

- Light Jackets and Blazers: A light jacket or blazer is ideal for layering during transitional weather. Look for jackets made from breathable materials like cotton or linen that provide enough warmth without making you too hot. A blazer can be layered over a maternity dress or tunic for a more polished look, while a light jacket can be paired with jeans or leggings for a casual outfit.

- Vests: A vest is another versatile layering piece that can add warmth without restricting your movement. Quilted vests, puffer vests, or fleece vests can be worn over long-sleeve tops or sweaters for an added layer of insulation. The sleeveless design makes vests perfect for transitional weather, as they allow your arms to move freely while still keeping your core warm.

The third trimester is a time of significant physical change, but with the right approach to fashion, you can feel both comfortable and stylish as you prepare for your baby's arrival. By prioritizing breathable, stretchy fabrics and maternity-specific designs, you can build a wardrobe that accommodates your growing belly without compromising on your personal style.

Maternity dresses, including empire waist, wrap, and maxi styles, offer the perfect balance of comfort and elegance, allowing you to dress for any occasion—whether it's a casual day out or a formal event. These styles provide the flexibility needed to grow with your body while flattering your bump in a way that makes you feel confident and radiant.

Layering is another essential aspect of third-trimester fashion, helping you stay comfortable in any weather. From lightweight cardigans and shawls for warm days to chunky sweaters and thermal layers for cold weather, layering techniques allow you to adjust your outfits to changing temperatures while maintaining comfort and ease of movement.

Ultimately, third-trimester fashion is about embracing your body's changes and finding ways to dress that make you feel confident, comfortable, and stylish. Whether you're heading to work, relaxing at home, or attending a special event, the right clothing choices will help you navigate the final months of pregnancy with grace and ease.

Postpartum Fashion

The postpartum period marks a significant transition for new mothers, not just emotionally and physically, but also in terms of fashion. After months of dressing to accommodate a growing baby bump, many women find themselves facing new challenges: adjusting to their postpartum body, navigating nursing, and prioritizing comfort while still wanting to look stylish. Postpartum fashion is about practicality and ease, but it doesn't have to be boring. With the right clothing choices, new mothers can feel confident, comfortable, and stylish as they embrace this new chapter of life.

In this chapter, we will explore how to transition from maternity wear to nursing and beyond, focusing on stylish and practical nursing wear, as well as the best Lounge-wear and active-wear options that offer comfort and functionality. By the end of this chapter, you will have a comprehensive guide to building a postpartum wardrobe that makes dressing easy, convenient, and enjoyable.

Transitioning from Maternity to Nursing and Beyond

After giving birth, many women find themselves in a transitional phase where their maternity clothes are too large, but pre-pregnancy clothes may not yet fit comfortably. The postpartum body is still adjusting, and it's important to find clothing that accommodates these changes while providing the comfort and support new mothers need, especially for breastfeeding.

1. Embracing Your Postpartum Body

It's essential to approach postpartum fashion with self-compassion and flexibility. The postpartum body is a reflection of the incredible process of carrying and delivering a baby, and it will take time for your body to recover and adjust. During this period, comfort should be your primary focus, and your wardrobe should help you feel both confident and at ease.

- Loose, Flowing Clothing: Loose-fitting clothing is ideal for the postpartum phase, as it provides room for movement and helps conceal areas that are still recovering from pregnancy. Tunics, loose dresses, and oversize tops are perfect for this phase because they provide comfort without clinging to the body.

- Elastic Waistbands and Adjustable Fits: Just as during pregnancy, elastic waistbands and adjustable clothing are key in the postpartum period. Whether you're wearing pants, skirts, or dresses, look for styles with elastic waistbands that can accommodate your body as it changes.

- Prioritize Easy Access for Nursing: If you're breastfeeding, it's essential to choose clothes that make nursing convenient. Look for tops and dresses with nursing access, such as button-down fronts, wrap designs, or hidden panels, to make breastfeeding easier, whether you're at home or out in public.

2. Re-purposing Maternity Wear

Some maternity pieces can still be useful during the postpartum phase, particularly those designed with flexibility and nursing in mind. Instead of rushing to buy an entirely new wardrobe, you can re-purpose some of your maternity clothes to fit your postpartum needs.

- Maternity Leggings and Joggers: Maternity leggings and joggers with over-the-belly or adjustable waistbands are perfect for postpartum wear. They offer the flexibility and comfort needed as your body heals and adjusts, making them ideal for lounging at home or running errands.

- Wrap and Empire Waist Dresses: Dresses with wrap designs or empire waistlines are also great for the postpartum phase. The wrap feature provides easy access for nursing, while the empire waist allows the fabric to flow over your postpartum belly without feeling restrictive.

- Loose, Stretchy Tops: Many maternity tops, especially those made from soft, stretchy fabrics like jersey or modal, can still be worn postpartum. These tops provide a comfortable fit and make nursing convenient with their looser designs.

Stylish and Practical Nursing Wear

For new mothers who are breastfeeding, nursing wear is an essential part of the postpartum wardrobe. Nursing clothes are specifically designed to provide easy access for breastfeeding, without sacrificing style. Modern nursing wear is both functional and fashionable, allowing new mothers to feel comfortable and stylish while nursing their baby at home or in public.

1. Nursing Tops

Nursing tops are a staple in any postpartum wardrobe. These tops are designed with discreet openings, such as hidden panels, zippers, or snap closures, that allow for easy access to nurse your baby while still keeping you covered.

- Button-Down Shirts: Button-down shirts are one of the most practical and stylish options for nursing mothers. The button front allows for easy access, and these shirts can be dressed up or down depending on the occasion. Pair a button-down with maternity leggings or jeans for a casual look, or wear it tucked into a skirt for a more polished outfit.

- Wrap Tops: Wrap tops are another great option for nursing because they can be adjusted to provide easy access for breastfeeding. They also tend to be flattering for the postpartum figure, as they cinch at the waist and flow over the belly, offering a forgiving fit.

- Nursing Tanks: Nursing tanks are a versatile option that can be layered under sweaters, cardigans, or blazers. These tanks often have built-in nursing bras with clip-down straps, making them easy to use for breastfeeding while still providing support. Nursing tanks are great for both day and night, as they can be worn alone in warmer weather or as a base layer in colder months.

- Zippered Nursing Tops: Many modern nursing tops feature hidden zippers along the sides or under the bust, providing discreet access for breastfeeding. These tops often look like regular t-shirts or blouses, making them a stylish and functional choice for nursing mothers who want to maintain their pre-pregnancy style.

2. Nursing Dresses

Nursing dresses are designed with easy access for breastfeeding while maintaining a flattering silhouette. Whether you're attending a formal event, going to a family gathering, or just running errands, a nursing dress offers both style and convenience.

- Wrap Dresses: As with wrap tops, wrap dresses are a popular option for nursing mothers because they can be easily adjusted for breastfeeding. These dresses allow you to pull one side of the dress aside for easy access, while the wrap design flatters your waist and creates a beautiful silhouette.

- Button-Down Dresses: Button-down dresses offer the same nursing convenience as button-down tops, with the added elegance of a dress. These dresses can be casual or formal, depending on the fabric and design, and they provide a stylish yet practical option for nursing mothers.

- Empire Waist Nursing Dresses: Dresses with an empire waist and discreet nursing access are perfect for postpartum wear. The high waistline provides a flattering fit, while the hidden nursing panels or zippers allow for easy breastfeeding.

- Nursing-Friendly Maxi Dresses: Maxi dresses are a great option for both comfort and style. Many nursing maxi dresses feature hidden nursing access or wrap designs, making them easy to nurse in while still providing a flowing, flattering fit. Maxi dresses are versatile and can be worn for various occasions, from casual days to special events.

3. Nursing Bras

Comfortable, supportive nursing bras are a must-have for breastfeeding mothers. Nursing bras are designed to provide easy access for breastfeeding while offering the necessary support as your breasts change in size.

- Soft-Cup Nursing Bras: Soft-cup nursing bras are wire-free and made from soft, breathable fabrics like cotton or bamboo. These bras provide gentle support and are perfect for everyday wear or sleeping. The drop-down cups make it easy to nurse, and the soft fabric prevents irritation on sensitive skin.

- Underwire Nursing Bras: For mothers who prefer more structured support, underwire nursing bras are a good option. These bras provide extra lift and shape, while still featuring drop-down cups for breastfeeding. Look for underwire bras with flexible wires that are gentle on your body, especially during the early postpartum weeks.

- Nursing Sports Bras: If you're active or enjoy working out, nursing sports bras offer the support needed during physical activity while still allowing for easy nursing access. These bras often have clip-down cups and are made from moisture-wicking fabrics to keep you comfortable during exercise.

Lounge-wear and Active-wear: Comfort Meets Functionality

As a new mother, comfort is a top priority, especially during the postpartum recovery period. Whether you're spending time at home with your newborn or getting back into physical activity, having comfortable and functional Lounge-wear and active-wear is essential.

1. Postpartum Lounge-wear

Lounge-wear is an important part of your postpartum wardrobe, as it allows you to relax comfortably at home while still feeling put together. Postpartum Lounge-wear should be soft, stretchy, and easy to move in, offering both comfort and style for new mothers.

- Maternity Leggings and Joggers: Maternity leggings and joggers are perfect for lounging at home during the postpartum phase. Look for leggings with high, stretchy waistbands that offer gentle support to your postpartum belly. Joggers with elastic or drawstring waistbands are also great for relaxing at home or running errands.

- Nursing-Friendly Tops: Loose, stretchy tops with nursing access are ideal for lounging at home. Whether you prefer nursing tanks, button-downs, or soft t-shirts, these tops provide comfort while making breastfeeding easy and convenient.

- Robe and Pajama Sets: A comfortable robe and pajama set is a must-have for postpartum wear, especially during the early weeks when you're spending a lot of time resting and recovering. Look for robes made from soft, breathable fabrics like cotton or bamboo, which can be layered over nursing pajamas for added warmth and comfort.

2. Postpartum Active-wear

Many new mothers are eager to get back into physical activity after giving birth, but it's important to wear active-wear that accommodates your postpartum body. Postpartum active-wear should be supportive, flexible, and designed to fit your body as it changes during the recovery period.

- High-Waited Leggings: High-waited leggings are essential for postpartum workouts because they provide support to your core and abdomen. Look for leggings made from stretchy, moisture-wicking materials that offer both comfort and compression. The high waistband helps provide gentle support to your postpartum belly, making it easier to move while still feeling secure. Some postpartum leggings even feature built-in compression panels that help support your core as it heals, making them an excellent choice for new mothers who want to ease back into physical activity.

- Supportive Nursing Sports Bras: Nursing sports bras are essential for postpartum exercise, especially for breastfeeding mothers. These bras provide the necessary support for physical activity while still allowing for easy access when it's time to nurse. Look for bras made from moisture-wicking materials to keep you cool and dry, and ensure the fit provides ample support to your changing breast size. Some nursing sports bras feature clip-down cups, while others have stretchy panels that allow you to easily pull them aside when breastfeeding.

- Loose, Breathable Tops: When it comes to postpartum active-wear, it's important to wear tops that are loose, breathable, and comfortable. Look for tank tops, t-shirts, or long-sleeve shirts made from soft, lightweight fabrics that won't restrict your movement. Some postpartum active-wear tops also feature built-in nursing access, making it easy to transition from exercise to breastfeeding without needing to change.

- Layering for Outdoor Activities: If you're getting back into outdoor activities like walking, hiking, or jogging, layering is key to staying comfortable. Start with a nursing sports bra and high-waited leggings as your base, then layer with a moisture-wicking t-shirt or tank top. In cooler weather, add a lightweight, zip-up hoodie or jacket that provides warmth without restricting movement. Many postpartum jackets also have nursing-friendly features, such as zippered or pull-aside panels for easy access when you're on the go.

3. Comfortable Footwear for Lounge-wear and Active-wear

Footwear is another important aspect of postpartum fashion, especially when it comes to comfort and support. Whether you're lounging around the house or heading out for a workout, the right shoes can make a big difference in how you feel.

- Slip-On Sneakers: Slip-on sneakers are perfect for new mothers who want a stylish yet practical footwear option. These shoes are easy to put on without bending over—an important feature when carrying a newborn—and they provide the necessary support for everyday activities. Look for slip-on sneakers with cushioned insoles and arch support to ensure comfort, especially if your feet are still swollen after pregnancy.

- Supportive Sandals or Slides: For lounging around the house or running quick errands, supportive sandals or slides are a great option. Look for sandals with cushioned soles and adjustable straps to accommodate any swelling in your feet. Brands that specialize in orthotic sandals often have options that provide excellent arch support and comfort for postpartum feet.

- Athletic Shoes: If you're planning to engage in more vigorous postpartum activities, such as walking, jogging, or going to the gym, investing in a good pair of athletic shoes is essential. Choose shoes with shock-absorbing soles and plenty of support for your arches and ankles. Some athletic shoes also feature extra room in the toe box, which is helpful if your feet are still adjusting after pregnancy.

The postpartum period is a time of significant transition, both physically and emotionally, and having the right wardrobe can make a world of difference. Whether you're breastfeeding, recovering from childbirth, or getting back into physical activity, your clothing should support your new lifestyle, offering both practicality and style.

Transitioning from maternity wear to nursing and beyond requires thoughtful choices that accommodate your changing body while providing easy access for breastfeeding. From button-down shirts and wrap dresses to nursing tanks and bras, modern nursing wear combines functionality with fashion, allowing new mothers to feel comfortable and confident in their daily lives.

Lounge-wear and active-wear are also crucial components of a postpartum wardrobe, as they prioritize comfort without sacrificing functionality. High-waisted leggings, supportive nursing sports bras, and soft, breathable tops are perfect for new mothers who want to relax at home or get back into physical activity. Coupled with comfortable footwear, these pieces provide the flexibility and support needed during the postpartum recovery period.

Ultimately, postpartum fashion is about finding balance—embracing comfort and practicality while still feeling stylish and confident as you navigate this new phase of motherhood. With the right clothing choices, you can build a postpartum wardrobe that meets your needs, helps you feel your best, and makes your transition into life with your new baby as smooth and enjoyable as possible.

Maternity Work-wear Essentials

The journey of pregnancy often brings significant changes to various aspects of life, and work is no exception. For many expectant mothers, balancing comfort with professionalism becomes a top priority as their bodies change and their wardrobe needs evolve. Dressing for the office during pregnancy requires thoughtful consideration, especially when it comes to choosing clothes that offer both style and comfort, while adhering to the dress code of the workplace.

In this chapter, we'll explore how to build a maternity work-wear wardrobe that suits different professional environments, from business casual to more formal corporate settings. We'll also discuss how to find work-wear that adapts to your growing belly and keeps you comfortable throughout the day. By the end of this chapter, you'll have a comprehensive understanding of how to dress for work during pregnancy with confidence and ease.

Business Casual vs. Corporate Maternity Style

When dressing for work during pregnancy, the first thing to consider is your workplace's dress code. Whether your office follows a business casual or formal corporate dress code, there are maternity options that will allow you to feel comfortable, confident, and professional as your body changes.

1. Business Casual Maternity Style

In a business casual setting, there's more flexibility in your work wardrobe, allowing for a blend of comfort and style. Business casual attire often includes relaxed yet polished pieces, making it easier to incorporate maternity clothes that provide comfort while still looking appropriate for the office.

- Maternity Dresses: Dresses are a versatile and comfortable option for business casual settings. Look for dresses with an empire waist or wrap design, as these styles allow for growth and offer an elegant yet relaxed silhouette. A-line or shift dresses are also great choices, as they provide room for your growing bump while maintaining a professional appearance. Pair dresses with flats or low-heeled shoes for a comfortable, all-day wear.

- Maternity Trousers: Maternity trousers with an elastic or over-the-belly waistband are a must-have for business casual attire. Look for pants made from stretchy, breathable fabrics like cotton or a blend of cotton and spandex, which will provide comfort as your belly grows. Cropped trousers or slim-fit maternity pants can be paired with blouses, tunics, or blazers to create a polished look without compromising on comfort.

- Blouses and Tunics: Loose-fitting blouses and tunics are perfect for a business casual office. Look for tops made from lightweight, breathable fabrics that drape nicely over your bump. Tops with side ruching or adjustable ties will grow with your belly and ensure a flattering fit. Pair blouses with maternity trousers or leggings to create an effortlessly chic office look.

- Cardigans and Blazers: Layers are essential in a business casual environment. Cardigans and blazers can be easily thrown over dresses or tops to add a professional touch to your outfit. Opt for cardigans in neutral or solid colors, which can be mixed and matched with various outfits. Blazers with an open-front design or stretchy side panels will accommodate your growing belly while still looking sharp.

2. Corporate Maternity Style

For those working in a formal corporate environment, dressing for pregnancy may feel more restrictive, but it's still possible to find stylish and comfortable options that meet the demands of a more professional dress code. The key to corporate maternity style is to focus on tailored, structured pieces that offer both sophistication and comfort.

- Maternity Blazers: A well-fitting maternity blazer is a cornerstone of corporate maternity wear. Look for blazers with extra room around the belly or side panels that provide flexibility as your body grows. Opt for classic colors like black, navy, or gray, which can be paired with various other pieces to create a professional look. Blazers with a longer cut can also offer more coverage and balance your proportions.

- Maternity Dresses and Pencil Skirts: In a corporate setting, dresses and skirts are often the go-to option for many women. Maternity pencil skirts with an over-the-belly waistband provide a sleek, polished look while still allowing room for your growing bump. Pair them with button-down blouses or structured tops for a professional outfit. Maternity sheath dresses or wrap dresses made from stretchy, high-quality fabrics are also ideal for corporate environments. These dresses can be dressed up with a blazer or statement necklace for formal meetings or events.

- Maternity Trousers and Dress Pants: Tailored maternity trousers are essential in a corporate setting. Look for trousers with a high-waited, over-the-belly panel that offers both support and comfort. Pair these trousers with tailored blouses or button-down shirts to maintain a professional appearance. Fabrics like wool blends, ponte, or gabardine offer structure and polish, making them suitable for corporate environments.

- Button-Down Shirts and Structured Tops: For a corporate office, structured tops and button-down shirts are essential. Choose shirts made from lightweight, breathable fabrics that allow room for your bump. Some maternity brands offer button-down shirts with extra length in the front or side ruching to accommodate your growing belly while still looking polished. Pair these shirts with tailored trousers or skirts for a sharp, professional look.

Tips for Finding Maternity Work-wear that Grows with You

One of the biggest challenges in dressing for work during pregnancy is finding clothes that can grow with you as your body changes. Maternity work-wear should provide flexibility and comfort while still maintaining a professional appearance. Here are some tips for finding work-wear that adapts to your body throughout pregnancy:

1. Prioritize Stretchy, Breathable Fabrics

When shopping for maternity work-wear, it's important to choose fabrics that offer stretch and breath-ability. Natural fabrics like cotton, bamboo, and modal are great options because they are soft, breathable, and gentle on sensitive skin. Fabrics with a blend of spandex or elastane provide the necessary stretch to accommodate your growing belly without feeling restrictive.

- Jersey Knit: Jersey knit fabrics are ideal for maternity work-wear because they are soft, stretchy, and drape nicely over your bump. Look for dresses, tops, and skirts made from jersey knit, as they will provide the comfort and flexibility needed for long days at the office.

- Ponte Fabric: Ponte is a thicker, stretchy fabric that offers structure and support while still being comfortable. Ponte maternity trousers, skirts, and dresses are perfect for professional environments, as they maintain a polished look without sacrificing comfort.

- Lightweight Blends: Fabrics that combine natural fibers like cotton or bamboo with a small percentage of synthetic fibers like spandex or polyester offer the best of both worlds. These blends provide the stretch needed for a growing belly while maintaining a professional appearance.

2. Look for Adjustable and Versatile Pieces

Maternity work-wear should be versatile enough to grow with you from the early stages of pregnancy through to the third trimester. Investing in adjustable pieces, such as wrap dresses, tunics with ties, or skirts with elastic waistbands, ensures that your wardrobe will adapt as your body changes.

- Wrap Dresses and Tops: Wrap designs are among the most versatile options for maternity work-wear. The adjustable tie allows you to customize the fit as your belly grows, and the wrap style provides a flattering silhouette throughout pregnancy.

- Elastic Waistbands and Panels: Maternity trousers, skirts, and leggings with elastic waistbands or over-the-belly panels provide comfort and flexibility as your body changes. Look for pants with adjustable features that allow you to tighten or loosen the waistband as needed.

- Side Ruching: Many maternity tops and dresses feature side ruching, which allows the fabric to expand as your belly grows. This design not only provides extra room but also creates a flattering fit that hugs your curves in all the right places.

3. Invest in Quality Staples

Building a maternity work wardrobe doesn't mean you need to purchase an entirely new set of clothes. By investing in a few high-quality staples, you can create a versatile wardrobe that can be mixed and matched with your existing pieces.

- Maternity Blazer: A well-fitted maternity blazer is one of the best invest-ments for your work wardrobe. Look for blazers with stretchy side panels or an open-front design that can be worn throughout your pregnancy and even postpartum.

- Tailored Maternity Pants: Maternity pants are another essential item that will get a lot of wear during your pregnancy. Invest in a pair of tailored trousers in a neutral color like black, navy, or gray, as these can be paired with various tops to create different outfits.

- Versatile Dresses: A few high-quality maternity dresses in neutral or solid colors can be worn multiple times throughout your pregnancy. Choose dresses that can be dressed up with a blazer or accessories for formal events or worn on their own for a more casual office day.

4. Focus on Layers for Adaptability

Layering is key to maintaining comfort in a work environment, especially as your body temperature fluctuates during pregnancy. Having the right layers ensures that you can adjust your outfit as needed throughout the day, whether you're feeling too warm or chilly.

- Cardigans and Blazers: A lightweight cardigan or a maternity blazer can be layered over dresses, tops, or tunics for added warmth or professionalism. These layers are easy to remove if you start to feel warm, providing flexibility as your body temperature changes.

- Scarves and Shawls: In cooler months, a soft scarf or shawl can add both warmth and style to your outfit. Choose scarves made from lightweight materials like cotton or wool blends, which can be easily adjusted throughout the day.

Office-Appropriate Comfort Solutions

Comfort is a top priority during pregnancy, especially when you're spending long hours at the office. Fortunately, there are plenty of office-appropriate comfort solutions that will help you stay comfortable throughout the workday without compromising your professional appearance.

1. Comfortable Shoes

Swollen feet and ankles are common during pregnancy, especially in the later stages, so choosing comfortable shoes for the office is essential. While you may be used to wearing heels or more formal footwear, it's important to prioritize support and comfort to avoid additional strain on your feet, back, and legs.

- Low-Heeled or Flat Shoes: Look for stylish flats or low-heeled shoes that provide proper arch support. Ballet flats, loafers, or low wedges are great options that maintain a professional look while offering more comfort than high heels. Many brands offer stylish flat shoes with cushioned insoles and wider toe boxes, which can help accommodate any swelling in your feet.

- Supportive Insoles: If you're committed to wearing heels or need to maintain a specific formal shoe style, consider adding cushioned insoles to your shoes for added support and comfort. Gel insoles or orthotic inserts can help reduce pressure on your feet and provide better shock absorption, making it easier to stay on your feet during the workday.

- Slip-On Shoes: In later pregnancy, bending over to tie shoes can become challenging, so slip-on shoes are a convenient option for work. Loafers, mules, or slip-on flats are easy to put on and take off without compromising on style or professionalism.

2. Maternity Compression Wear

Swelling in the legs, feet, and ankles is common during pregnancy, particularly for women who spend a lot of time sitting or standing at work. Wearing maternity compression stockings or socks can help improve circulation and reduce swelling.

- Compression Stockings: These stockings are designed to gently compress the legs, improving blood flow and helping to prevent varicose veins, swelling, and discomfort. Maternity compression stockings come in a variety of styles, from knee-highs to full-length tights, and can be worn under trousers, skirts, or dresses for a discreet solution to swelling.

- Maternity Tights: If you work in a more formal setting where skirts or dresses are part of your wardrobe, maternity tights are a great option. These tights offer gentle compression and often feature a supportive panel that fits over your belly, providing both comfort and style. Look for tights made from breathable, stretchy fabrics that accommodate your changing shape.

3. Belly Bands and Support Belts

As your belly grows, you may experience added pressure on your lower back and pelvis, making sitting for long periods or standing during work uncomfortable. A belly band or maternity support belt can provide much-needed relief by offering support to your belly and lower back.

- Belly Bands: Belly bands are stretchy fabric bands worn around your midsection to provide gentle support to your lower back and abdomen. They help take the pressure off your pelvis and can be worn discreetly under your work clothes. Many belly bands are designed to fit over the top of your maternity trousers or skirts, providing extra support and helping to keep your pants in place.

- Maternity Support Belts: For women experiencing more significant discomfort, maternity support belts offer additional support to the lower back and pelvis. These belts are adjustable and provide firmer support than a belly band, making them ideal for women who spend a lot of time on their feet. Support belts can also help improve posture, reducing strain on the back and shoulders.

4. Office-Appropriate Lounge-wear Options

In more relaxed work environments or for those working from home during pregnancy, office-appropriate Lounge-wear is a comfortable yet stylish option. Lounge-wear can be both professional and comfortable, especially when you choose pieces made from soft, breathable fabrics that offer a relaxed fit without looking too casual.

- Maternity Joggers and Knit Pants: Maternity joggers or knit pants are perfect for working in a business casual or remote work environment. Look for joggers made from high-quality fabrics like ponte or jersey, which offer a more structured look while still feeling incredibly comfortable. Pair these pants with a loose-fitting blouse or sweater for a professional yet relaxed office look.

- Tunic Sweaters and Cardigans: Tunic sweaters or cardigans made from soft knit fabrics are comfortable enough for lounging but polished enough for a professional setting. Tunics can be paired with leggings, maternity trousers, or knit pants to create a stylish, office-appropriate outfit that still prioritizes comfort.

- Maternity Blouses and T-Shirts: Soft, stretchy maternity blouses or t-shirts in neutral or solid colors can be dressed up with a blazer or cardigan for a more professional look. These tops offer both comfort and style, making them ideal for days when you want to prioritize comfort without sacrificing your polished appearance.

Dressing for work during pregnancy doesn't have to be a challenge. With the right combination of maternity work-wear essentials, you can create a wardrobe that grows with you, providing both comfort and style throughout your pregnancy. Whether you work in a business casual environment or a more formal corporate office, there are plenty of options available to help you maintain a professional appearance while staying comfortable.

By choosing stretchy, breathable fabrics, investing in versatile and adjustable pieces, and incorporating layers and supportive accessories, you can build a maternity work wardrobe that meets the demands of your changing body. Comfortable footwear, compression wear, and belly support solutions further ensure that you stay comfortable during long hours at the office.

Ultimately, maternity work-wear is about finding the balance between comfort, practicality, and professionalism. With thoughtful choices, you can navigate your pregnancy with confidence, knowing that your wardrobe is working with you every step of the way. Whether you're attending meetings, working from home, or navigating the daily grind, the right maternity work-wear will help you feel empowered and ready to tackle any professional challenge.

Dressing for Parties, Weddings, and Social Events

The experience of pregnancy brings a lot of exciting milestones, and with them come numerous social gatherings and special occasions. Whether you're attending a wedding, a holiday party, or even your own baby shower or gender reveal, dressing for these events while pregnant presents a unique challenge: How can you balance comfort, accommodate your growing bump, and still feel glamorous? Fortunately, maternity fashion has come a long way, and today's maternity formal wear options are designed with both style and comfort in mind.

In this chapter, we will explore how to find glamorous maternity formal wear that doesn't sacrifice comfort, offer tips on styling your bump for various celebrations and events, and provide dress ideas for baby showers, gender reveals, and maternity photo-shoots. By the end of this chapter, you'll have a comprehensive guide to looking and feeling your best at every event, regardless of your stage of pregnancy.

Maternity Formal Wear: Finding Glamour with Comfort

Attending formal events while pregnant can be a daunting task. Whether it's a black-tie wedding, a gala, or a fancy holiday party, many women worry that maternity wear won't provide the elegance and style needed for such occasions. However, maternity fashion has evolved to offer a range of options that combine glamour and comfort, ensuring that pregnant women can feel confident and chic at any formal event.

1. Prioritize Comfort and Flexibility

When choosing maternity formal wear, comfort should always be a top priority. Formal events often last several hours, so it's essential to find clothing that allows you to move freely, sit comfortably, and accommodate any physical changes. The key is to look for maternity dresses made from stretchy, breathable fabrics that provide flexibility while still offering a polished appearance.

- Jersey Knit and Stretch Fabrics: Many maternity formal dresses are made from jersey knit, a stretchy and soft fabric that drapes beautifully over your bump without feeling restrictive. Stretch fabrics, such as elastane blends, allow for movement and growth, ensuring that your dress fits comfortably throughout the event.

- Adjustable Designs: Dresses with adjustable features, like wrap dresses or empire waist styles, offer both comfort and adaptability. Wrap dresses, for example, allow you to adjust the fit as your belly grows, while empire waist dresses emphasize your bust and flow elegantly over your bump.

- Breathable Fabrics: Pregnancy can cause you to feel warmer than usual, especially in formal settings where multiple layers or heavy fabrics might be involved. Look for dresses made from breathable fabrics like cotton blends or lightweight chiffon, which will keep you cool and comfortable throughout the event.

2. Embrace Glamorous Details

Even though comfort is key, that doesn't mean you have to sacrifice glamour. Many maternity dresses feature beautiful detailing that adds elegance to your look, allowing you to feel stylish and polished at formal events.

- Embellishments and Sequins: Dresses with subtle embellishments, sequins, or beading can add a touch of glamour without overwhelming your look. Sequined bodices or embellishments along the neckline or waist can elevate a simple dress into something suitable for a formal occasion.

- Lace and Chiffon: Lace overlays and chiffon skirts add a delicate, feminine touch to maternity formal wear. These lightweight fabrics create a flowing, elegant silhouette that flatters your bump while remaining comfortable. Dresses with lace detailing on the sleeves, back, or bodice are particularly popular for formal events like weddings.

- Elegant Draping: Draped designs are often used in maternity formal wear to create soft, flattering lines that highlight your bump while maintaining a sophisticated appearance. Whether it's a draped bodice, a cascading chiffon overlay, or pleated detailing, these styles provide a sense of luxury while ensuring comfort.

3. The Right Fit for Each Stage of Pregnancy

As your body changes throughout pregnancy, your clothing needs will also change. When shopping for maternity formal wear, consider the specific stage of pregnancy you'll be in during the event, and choose a dress that will accommodate those changes.

- Early Pregnancy: In the earlier stages of pregnancy, your bump may not be very pronounced, so you have more flexibility with styles. Wrap dresses, empire waistlines, and flowy A-line dresses are excellent choices, as they can transition with you as your belly grows.

- Mid-Pregnancy: During the second trimester, your bump will be more visible, and this is a great time to embrace styles that show off your pregnancy. Body-con dresses made from stretchy fabric or fitted dresses with ruching can highlight your bump in a flattering way while still being comfortable.

- Late Pregnancy: In the third trimester, your belly is at its fullest, and you'll want to prioritize comfort above all else. Look for dresses with plenty of room for your bump, such as empire waist gowns, maxi dresses, or loose, flowing styles made from stretchy, breathable fabrics.

Styling Your Bump for Celebrations and Special Occasions

Whether you're attending a formal wedding or a casual family gathering, styling your bump for social events can be a fun and rewarding experience. With the right approach, you can create looks that are not only comfortable but also stylish, allowing you to enjoy the occasion feeling confident and beautiful.

1. Emphasize Your Bump with Flattering Silhouettes

The key to dressing for any special occasion during pregnancy is to find silhouettes that flatter your bump. Rather than trying to hide your pregnancy, embrace it with styles that accentuate your curves in a beautiful way.

- Empire Waist Dresses: Empire waist dresses are universally flattering for pregnant women. The high waistline sits just below the bust, drawing attention to your upper body while allowing the fabric to flow freely over your belly. This style is perfect for both casual and formal occasions, as it provides comfort without compromising on style.

- Body-con Dresses: If you want to showcase your bump, a body con dress is a fantastic option. Body-con dresses are made from stretchy, figure-hugging fabrics that accentuate your curves and highlight your belly. These dresses are great for events where you want to make a statement and celebrate your pregnancy.

- Maxi Dresses: Maxi dresses are ideal for outdoor events or summer celebrations. Their long, flowing design offers plenty of room for your bump, while their casual elegance makes them suitable for both formal and informal gatherings. Choose maxi dresses made from lightweight fabrics like chiffon or jersey for maximum comfort and style.

2. Accessories to Elevate Your Look

Accessories play a crucial role in elevating your maternity look and adding a touch of glamour to any outfit. When dressing for a special occasion, choose accessories that complement your dress while enhancing your overall look.

- Statement Jewelry: Bold, statement jewelry can transform a simple maternity dress into a show-stopping outfit. Whether it's a chunky necklace, oversize earrings, or a statement bracelet, jewelry adds an element of elegance and sophistication to your ensemble.

- Belts and Sashes: Belts and sashes worn above your bump can create a more defined silhouette and draw attention to your waistline. Opt for a decorative belt with embellishments or a simple ribbon sash in a contrasting color to add visual interest to your dress.

- Shoes: Comfortable shoes are essential when dressing for a social event during pregnancy. While you may want to wear heels for a more formal look, consider low block heels or wedges, which provide more support than stilettos. If you prefer flats, look for embellished ballet flats or sandals with supportive insoles to ensure comfort throughout the event.

3. Hair and Makeup to Complete the Look

Your hair and makeup can also enhance your maternity style, helping you feel polished and put-together for any celebration. Whether you prefer a more natural look or want to go all out with glamorous makeup, choose styles that reflect your personality while complementing your outfit.

- Soft Waves or Updos: Soft waves, curls, or romantic updos are popular choices for formal events. These hairstyles are elegant without being overly fussy, and they can help balance out your outfit, especially if you're wearing a flowy dress or gown.

- Fresh, Glowing Makeup: Pregnancy often brings a natural glow, so embrace it with fresh, radiant makeup. A luminous foundation or BB cream paired with soft blush and highlighter will enhance your skin's natural radiance. If you're attending a formal event, you can add a pop of color with bold lips or smoky eyes for a more dramatic look.

Dress Ideas for Baby Showers, Gender Reveals, and Photo-shoots

Pregnancy is full of exciting milestones, and some of the most memorable events are your baby shower, gender reveal party, and maternity photo shoot. These are occasions where you'll want to look and feel your best, and the right outfit can help make these moments even more special.

1. Baby Shower Dresses

Your baby shower is a time to celebrate your pregnancy with family and friends, so finding the perfect dress is essential. When choosing a dress for your baby shower, consider the theme, venue, and season, as well as your personal style and comfort.

- Floral Maxi Dresses: Floral prints are a popular choice for baby showers, as they exude femininity and joy. A floral maxi dress made from lightweight chiffon or jersey fabric is perfect for an outdoor or springtime shower, offering both elegance and comfort.

- Lace Dresses: Lace dresses are another classic option for baby showers. The delicate texture of lace adds a touch of romance to your outfit, making it ideal for more formal or indoor events. Choose a dress with lace detailing along the bodice, sleeves, or hemline for a timeless, elegant look.

- Pastel Colors: Many women opt for pastel-colored dresses for their baby shower, as these soft hues create a sense of warmth and serenity. Shades like blush pink, lavender, sky blue, and mint green are especially popular for baby showers. These colors can also subtly hint at the baby's gender if that's something you want to share or celebrate during the event. Opt for a flowing, comfortable dress that allows you to move easily and feel relaxed while enjoying your special day.

2. Gender Reveal Dresses

Gender reveal parties are another fun milestone during pregnancy, where many couples share the news of their baby's gender with family and friends. Your outfit for this occasion can reflect the exciting theme, and there are various playful and stylish ways to dress for the event.

- Split Color Dresses: A trendy option for gender reveals is a dress that features both pink and blue. Some dresses are designed with one half in pink and the other in blue, creating a perfect nod to the gender reveal theme. It's a fun and fashionable way to play into the event while keeping the big secret until the big moment.

- Flowy, White Dresses: A white dress is a great neutral choice for a gender reveal party, especially if the reveal itself involves colorful elements like balloons, confetti, or smoke. A white maxi dress or midi dress creates a fresh, clean canvas that allows the reveals colors to stand out even more. Pair it with simple accessories and let the gender reveal be the highlight.

- Pastel or Neutral Tones: If you prefer a softer approach, dresses in neutral or pastel tones can also work well for gender reveal parties. Soft pink, baby blue, or light beige dresses complement the theme without being too obvious. Flowing fabrics, like chiffon or tulle, can add an ethereal quality to your outfit, making it both comfortable and stylish for the occasion.

3. Maternity Photo-shoot Dresses

A maternity photo shoot is a once-in-a-lifetime experience where you get to capture the beauty and joy of your pregnancy. Finding the right outfit for this special moment is key, as it will help you feel confident and radiant while creating memories to cherish forever.

- Fitted, Stretchy Dresses: Fitted maternity dresses that highlight your bump are perfect for showcasing your pregnancy in photos. A body-hugging dress made from soft, stretchy fabric like jersey or modal can create a striking silhouette, capturing the natural curves of your body. Choose solid colors like white, navy, or burgundy for a clean, timeless look that won't distract from the focus on you and your bump.

- Flowy, Maxi Dresses with Draping: Flowing maxi dresses with long, draping fabric create a sense of movement and elegance in photos. Dresses with chiffon or tulle skirts that flow in the breeze can add a dreamy, ethereal quality to your photo shoot. Many women opt for off-the-shoulder or sleeveless maxi dresses, as these styles allow for beautiful arm and shoulder shots while emphasizing the natural beauty of pregnancy.

- Goddess-Inspired Dresses: A popular trend for maternity photo-shoots is goddess-inspired dresses, often featuring long, flowing trains or capes. These dresses add a regal and majestic vibe to your photos, elevating the maternity shoot to something truly special. Dresses with a plunging neckline, delicate lace details, or a dramatic train create a goddess-like appearance, perfect for capturing the strength and grace of pregnancy.

- Bohemian Styles: For a more laid-back and earthy look, bohemian-style dresses are a great choice for maternity photo-shoots. Dresses with crochet details, bell sleeves, or vintage-inspired lace evoke a free-spirited, natural vibe. Opt for neutral colors like cream, ivory, or light pastels to keep the focus on your connection with nature and the beauty of your pregnancy.

4. Practical Tips for Photo-shoot Dressing

- Comfort is Key: Even though a maternity photo shoot is a special occasion, comfort should still be a priority. Make sure the dress you choose allows you to move freely and doesn't restrict your movement or breathing, especially as photo-shoots can take time.

- Consider the Location: The location of your photo shoot will play a role in the type of dress you choose. For outdoor shoots, long, flowing dresses work beautifully against natural backdrops like fields, beaches, or forests. If your photo shoot takes place indoors or in a more urban setting, a fitted dress or something more structured might suit the environment better.

- Accessorize Wisely: Keep accessories simple for maternity photo-shoots, as the focus should be on you and your bump. A delicate necklace, a floral crown, or a simple pair of earrings can enhance your look without overwhelming it. If your dress has a dramatic neckline or back, consider wearing your hair up to highlight these features.

Pregnancy is filled with moments worth celebrating, and each special occasion presents an opportunity to showcase your style while embracing the beauty of your growing bump. From glamorous formal events to intimate gatherings like baby showers and maternity photo-shoots, dressing for these occasions doesn't mean sacrificing comfort. In fact, today's maternity fashion has evolved to provide a wide range of elegant, flattering, and comfortable options for every event.

Whether you're attending a wedding, enjoying a family gathering, or hosting your own gender reveal or baby shower, the right maternity outfit can help you feel confident, beautiful, and comfortable. Prioritize fabrics and designs that offer flexibility and breath-ability, while also selecting styles that flatter your bump and reflect your personal taste. From empire waist dresses and maxi gowns to fitted body con styles, there's a perfect look for every celebration.

By choosing the right silhouettes, accessorizing wisely, and embracing maternity fashion that combines glamour with practicality, you can enjoy every special moment during your pregnancy feeling like the best version of yourself. The key is to embrace your pregnancy, have fun with your fashion choices, and focus on outfits that make you feel comfortable, confident, and ready to celebrate each milestone along the way.

Staying Active: Maternity Sportswear

Staying active during pregnancy is incredibly beneficial for both physical and mental well-being. Regular exercise helps reduce common pregnancy discomforts, such as back pain and fatigue, and promotes better sleep, improved mood, and even an easier labor. However, as your body changes, so do your workout needs—particularly when it comes to clothing. Maternity sportswear should offer the flexibility, support, and comfort necessary for active moms-to-be, while also accommodating the growing belly, changes in body temperature, and increased sensitivity in areas like the breasts and back.

This chapter will cover how to find maternity active-wear for various forms of exercise, including yoga, walking, and gym workouts. We'll also explore comfortable footwear options for active moms-to-be, as well as maternity swimwear and beachwear tips for staying active in the water. By the end of this chapter, you'll have a thorough understanding of how to stay comfortable and stylish while keeping up with your fitness routine during pregnancy.

Finding Maternity Active-wear for Yoga, Walking, and Gym Workouts

Exercising during pregnancy, whether it's through yoga, walking, or gym workouts, requires the right type of clothing to ensure you stay comfortable, supported, and flexible. The right maternity active-wear should move with your body, offer proper ventilation, and provide the necessary support for your changing shape. Many pregnant women struggle with finding workout clothes that grow with their bump, but fortunately, maternity active-wear brands now offer a range of stylish, functional, and comfortable options.

1. Maternity Yoga Wear

Prenatal yoga is one of the most popular forms of exercise during pregnancy, offering numerous benefits such as increased flexibility, improved circulation, and reduced stress. The key to yoga wear during pregnancy is flexibility and breath-ability, as yoga requires a wide range of movements and poses. Maternity yoga wear should allow for free movement without restricting your belly, hips, or legs.

- Stretchy Leggings: Maternity yoga leggings are a must-have for any yoga practice. Look for leggings made from soft, stretchy fabrics like spandex or modal, which provide flexibility and room for your growing belly. High-waited maternity leggings with an over-the-bump panel offer gentle support to your abdomen and lower back, keeping you comfortable during stretching and bending poses. Many maternity leggings are also made with moisture-wicking materials to keep you cool and dry during your practice.

- Breathable Yoga Tops: A breathable, stretchy top is essential for prenatal yoga. Look for maternity yoga tops that provide plenty of room for your bump and offer enough coverage during poses like downward dog. Tops with side ruching or extra length are ideal, as they can grow with your belly while providing coverage. For added support, choose tops with built-in bras or racer back designs, which help support the bust during yoga movements.

- Supportive Sports Bras: As your breasts grow during pregnancy, finding a supportive sports bra becomes essential, especially for yoga. Look for maternity sports bras that offer soft, wireless support and adjustable straps, allowing you to customize the fit as your body changes. A bra made from moisture-wicking fabric is ideal, as it will keep you cool and comfortable during longer sessions.

2. Maternity Active-wear for Walking

Walking is one of the easiest and most effective ways to stay active during pregnancy. It's low-impact, doesn't require any special equipment, and can be done at your own pace. The key to dressing for walking during pregnancy is to find clothes that offer support, regulate your body temperature, and allow for easy movement.

- Loose-Fitting Maternity T-Shirts: When walking, it's important to wear a breathable, loose-fitting t-shirt or tank top that allows air to circulate and keeps you cool. Maternity t-shirts made from moisture-wicking fabrics like polyester blends or bamboo are perfect for walking, as they help regulate your body temperature and prevent overheating. Look for tops with extra length to cover your belly, or shirts with side ruching that allow room for growth.

- Comfortable Maternity Joggers: For outdoor walking or cooler weather, maternity joggers or sweatpants provide both comfort and style. Look for pants with an adjustable waistband or over-the-belly support that offer gentle compression and support. Maternity joggers made from breathable fabrics like cotton or a cotton-spandex blend offer the flexibility you need while walking, and they can easily be paired with a lightweight jacket or hoodie.

- Lightweight Maternity Jackets: If you're walking outdoors, a lightweight jacket or hoodie is essential, especially during cooler weather or early mornings. Maternity jackets with adjustable side panels or drawstrings can grow with your bump, offering comfort and warmth without feeling too tight or restrictive.

3. Maternity Gym Wear

For pregnant women who enjoy more intense workouts at the gym, such as weight lifting, cycling, or cardio, it's important to find active-wear that offers both flexibility and support. Maternity gym wear should allow for full range of motion, while also providing the necessary coverage and support for your growing belly and bust.

- High-Support Sports Bras: During gym workouts, you'll need a sports bra that offers high support, especially as your breasts grow during pregnancy. Look for bras with wide, adjustable straps and a wide band under the bust for extra support. Maternity sports bras made from moisture-wicking fabric are ideal for high-intensity workouts, as they help keep you cool and prevent chafing.

- Maternity Tank Tops: A comfortable, stretchy tank top is a staple for gym workouts during pregnancy. Look for tops with built-in bras or racer back designs that offer support and keep you cool. Maternity tanks with extra length and side ruching are perfect for gym workouts, as they allow room for your growing belly while ensuring coverage during exercises like squats or lunges.

- Compression Leggings: Maternity compression leggings provide the support needed for gym workouts while also helping to reduce swelling in the legs and improve circulation. These leggings often feature an over-the-bump panel that offers gentle compression to your belly and lower back, helping to relieve pressure during workouts. Compression leggings made from moisture-wicking materials are ideal for cardio or high-intensity training, as they keep you cool and dry.

Comfortable Footwear for Active Moms-to-Be

One of the most important aspects of staying active during pregnancy is finding the right footwear. Your feet may swell, your center of gravity may shift, and your joints may become more sensitive during pregnancy, making proper footwear essential for comfort and safety.

1. Supportive Sneakers

When it comes to walking, jogging, or gym workouts, supportive sneakers are essential for pregnant women. Look for sneakers that offer cushioned soles, arch support, and breathable materials. As your body weight increases, your feet may experience more pressure, so finding shoes with adequate support is crucial for preventing foot pain, back pain, and joint discomfort.

- Arch Support and Cushioning: Look for sneakers with ample arch support and cushioned soles, which help absorb shock and reduce pressure on your feet. Many pregnant women find that their arches flatten during pregnancy, so extra support is essential for maintaining good posture and preventing discomfort.

- Breathable and Lightweight: Choose sneakers made from breathable mesh or moisture-wicking materials to keep your feet cool and dry during workouts. Lightweight shoes are easier on your feet and legs, allowing for more comfortable movement during exercise.

- Slip-On Sneakers: As your belly grows, bending over to tie your shoes may become more difficult. Slip-on sneakers or shoes with elastic laces are a convenient option for active moms-to-be. These shoes provide the support you need without the hassle of laces, making them easier to put on and take off.

2. Sandals and Slip-On Shoes

For casual walking or light outdoor activities, sandals and slip-on shoes can be a comfortable alternative to sneakers. Look for shoes that provide enough support and cushioning to prevent foot pain or swelling.

- Supportive Sandals: Many sandals offer arch support and cushioned soles, making them a great option for walking during the warmer months. Look for sandals with adjustable straps, as your feet may swell during pregnancy. Brands that specialize in orthotic sandals offer styles that provide excellent support and comfort while still looking stylish.

- Slip-On Shoes with Cushioned Insoles: If you're looking for a more casual option for walking or light exercise, slip-on shoes with cushioned insoles are a great choice. These shoes are easy to put on and take off, and they provide comfort and support for your feet during pregnancy.

3. Compression Socks

Swelling in the legs, ankles, and feet is common during pregnancy, especially after long walks or standing for extended periods. Compression socks can help reduce swelling and improve circulation, making them a great addition to your active-wear wardrobe.

- Maternity Compression Socks: Maternity compression socks are designed to provide gentle compression to your legs and feet, helping to reduce swelling and discomfort. These socks are perfect for wearing during walks, gym workouts, or even while traveling. Look for socks that offer graduated compression, which means the pressure is higher at the ankles and gradually decreases up the leg.

- Moisture-Wicking Compression Socks: If you're staying active in warmer weather, moisture-wicking compression socks are a great option. These socks help keep your feet cool and dry while providing the necessary compression to reduce swelling.

Maternity Swimwear and Beachwear Tips

Swimming is one of the most effective low-impact exercises for pregnant women, offering numerous benefits such as reduced joint pain, improved circulation, and stress relief. Whether you're taking a dip in the pool for exercise or lounging on the beach during a tropical getaway, finding the right maternity swimwear is essential for staying comfortable and stylish.

1. Maternity Swimsuits

Maternity swimsuits are designed to accommodate your growing belly and provide support where you need it most. Whether you're swimming for exercise or simply relaxing at the beach, a well-fitting maternity swimsuit can make all the difference. There are several styles available, so it's essential to choose one that suits your body shape, stage of pregnancy, and personal comfort preferences.

1.1 One-Piece Maternity Swimsuits

One-piece swimsuits are a popular option for pregnant women because they offer full coverage and support. Many maternity one-pieces come with extra features such as built-in belly panels, adjustable straps, and padded cups to provide extra support to your growing bust and belly.

- Ruching for Flexibility: One-piece maternity swimsuits often feature ruching along the sides, which allows the fabric to stretch as your belly grows. This gives you a comfortable fit throughout your pregnancy, as the ruching provides extra room for your bump without feeling too tight.

- Built-In Support: Look for swimsuits with built-in bras or bust support, which are essential during pregnancy as your breasts grow and may become more sensitive. Adjustable straps are also important for ensuring a comfortable and secure fit, especially as your body changes.

1.2 Maternity Bikinis and Tankinis

If you prefer more flexibility or want to showcase your bump, maternity bikinis and tankinis are excellent options. These two-piece swimsuits offer more versatility, as you can mix and match tops and bottoms to create the perfect fit.

- Maternity Bikinis: Maternity bikinis are designed with adjustable features to accommodate your changing body. The bottoms typically have a higher waistband to sit comfortably over or below your bump, while the tops offer extra coverage and support. Halter-style bikini tops with adjustable ties are great for pregnant women, as they provide the flexibility to tighten or loosen the fit as needed.

- Tankinis for More Coverage: For moms-to-be who want more coverage but still like the flexibility of a two-piece swimsuit, tankinis are the perfect solution. The longer top covers your bump, while the separate bottoms offer ease of movement. Tankinis often have adjustable ties on the sides to allow for a customized fit, and they provide more comfort for women who prefer not to wear a one-piece.

1.3 Swim Dresses and Maternity Cover-Ups

For women who want more coverage or prefer a more modest look, maternity swim dresses and cover-ups offer a stylish and practical solution. Swim dresses have built-in swimsuits underneath, providing coverage while still allowing you to swim comfortably.

- Swim Dresses for Elegance and Comfort: Maternity swim dresses are great for women who prefer a bit more coverage while still enjoying time at the beach or pool. These dresses provide a feminine, elegant look while still being functional for swimming. They often feature built-in bust support and extra room around the belly to ensure a comfortable fit.

- Lightweight Cover-Ups: If you're spending a day at the beach or pool, a lightweight cover-up is a must. Look for cover-ups made from breathable, quick-drying fabrics like cotton or linen, which provide sun protection while still keeping you cool. Flowy kaftans, sarongs, or tunics are great options for easy layering over your swimsuit and can also double as stylish outfits for post-swim lounging.

2. Maternity Beachwear Tips

Staying active at the beach while pregnant requires more than just finding the right swimsuit. You'll want to ensure that you're protected from the sun, staying hydrated, and comfortable as you enjoy outdoor activities.

- Sun Protection: Pregnancy can make your skin more sensitive, so it's crucial to prioritize sun protection. Look for swimwear and beachwear with built-in UPF (Ultraviolet Protection Factor) for extra protection from harmful UV rays. Always wear a wide-brimmed hat and use pregnancy-safe sunscreen to protect your skin from sunburn.

- Hydration: Staying hydrated is especially important during pregnancy, especially when you're spending time outdoors in the sun. Bring plenty of water with you and take breaks in the shade to avoid overheating. It's also a good idea to have light snacks on hand to keep your energy levels up.

- Comfortable Footwear for the Beach: If you're walking on the beach, opt for comfortable sandals or flip-flops with good arch support. Avoid overly flat shoes, which can put extra strain on your back and feet. Sandals with cushioned soles and adjustable straps are ideal for providing the support you need while still being practical for sandy terrain.

3. Active Swimwear for Water Workouts

Many pregnant women enjoy swimming or water aerobics as part of their prenatal exercise routine. These low-impact exercises help relieve joint pressure and improve circulation while providing a full-body workout that's safe and gentle on your body. When choosing swimwear for water workouts, prioritize comfort, support, and functionality.

- High-Support Swim Tops: For water workouts, you'll need a swimsuit that offers more support than your typical beachwear. Look for swim tops with built-in bras or extra bust support, as well as adjustable straps that allow you to customize the fit.

- Full-Coverage Bottoms: Whether you prefer a one-piece or a two-piece, make sure your swim bottoms offer full coverage and stay in place during exercise. High-waited bottoms or swim shorts are great options for water workouts, as they provide the support you need without riding up or feeling too loose.

- Chlorine-Resistant Fabrics: If you're swimming regularly in a chlorinated pool, look for maternity swimwear made from chlorine-resistant fabrics. These materials are designed to withstand the harsh effects of chlorine and will last longer, making them ideal for frequent swimmers.

Staying active during pregnancy is one of the best ways to support your physical and emotional well-being, and with the right maternity sportswear, you can maintain your fitness routine comfortably and confidently. Whether you're practicing prenatal yoga, walking, swimming, or hitting the gym, your maternity active-wear should provide the flexibility, support, and breathability you need to accommodate your growing body.

From stretchy, moisture-wicking leggings to high-support sports bras and breathable tops, maternity active-wear is designed to move with you and ensure that you stay comfortable throughout your workouts. Proper footwear is also essential, with supportive sneakers and sandals offering the necessary arch support and cushioning for active moms-to-be.

In addition to land-based exercises, maternity swimwear offers pregnant women a comfortable and stylish way to stay active in the water. Whether you prefer a one-piece, bikini, or swim dress, there are plenty of options to suit your style while providing the support and comfort needed during water workouts or a relaxing day at the beach.

Ultimately, staying active during pregnancy is about finding the right balance between comfort, support, and style. With the proper maternity sportswear, you'll be able to enjoy all the benefits of physical activity while feeling confident and comfortable in your clothing.

Footwear That Supports Pregnancy

Pregnancy brings a host of changes to a woman's body, and some of the most common physical discomforts occur in the feet. As your pregnancy progresses, the additional weight, hormonal changes, and fluid retention can cause swelling, aches, and even changes in foot size. With these transformations, finding the right footwear becomes essential not only for comfort but also for overall health. Improper shoes can exacerbate discomfort, leading to more serious issues like back pain, joint pain, and poor posture.

In this chapter, we'll explore the importance of comfortable shoes during pregnancy, go over various stylish yet functional footwear options—ranging from flats to sneakers to sandals—and provide tips for choosing maternity-specific footwear that supports your evolving needs. By the end of this chapter, you will have a solid understanding of how to select footwear that complements your pregnancy journey while keeping you stylish and comfortable.

The Importance of Comfortable Shoes During Pregnancy

The demands of pregnancy can put significant pressure on your feet, altering not only how you walk but also how your body distributes weight. These changes affect your balance, posture, and overall comfort. By choosing the right footwear, you can ease the physical stress that comes with pregnancy and ensure that you are fully supported as your body changes.

1. Swelling and Foot Pain

One of the most common foot-related issues during pregnancy is swelling, or edema, especially in the third trimester. Edema often occurs because your body retains more fluids during pregnancy, and gravity causes this excess fluid to pool in your lower extremities. This can make your feet feel tight, sore, and uncomfortable, particularly if you're on your feet for long periods or wearing shoes that are too tight.

Proper footwear during pregnancy can help alleviate swelling by allowing your feet to breathe and providing enough space for slight increases in foot size. Footwear with adjustable straps or laces can be loosened to accommodate swelling, ensuring that your shoes never pinch or restrict your feet.

2. Shifting Center of Gravity and Balance

As your baby bump grows, your center of gravity shifts, and this affects how you walk and balance. The shift in your center of gravity causes you to lean back more, which can lead to a condition called lordosis, or an exaggerated inward curve of the lower back. This postural change places additional stress on your feet, ankles, and lower back.

Wearing footwear with proper arch support and cushioning can help you maintain balance and relieve some of the pressure on your lower back and legs. Shoes with a wide base or lower heels are also beneficial for preventing falls, as your balance may be compromised as your belly grows.

3. Changes in Foot Size and Shape

Hormonal changes during pregnancy can lead to relaxation of the ligaments in your body, including those in your feet. This may cause your feet to spread or flatten, leading to an increase in shoe size. It's not uncommon for women to experience an increase of half a size to a full size during pregnancy, and for some, this change can be permanent.

Choosing shoes with flexibility or a wider fit is essential during pregnancy, as it allows your feet to expand without causing discomfort. Shoes that are too tight can worsen foot pain and lead to other issues like blisters or bunions.

4. Preventing Back, Hip, and Joint Pain

In addition to foot discomfort, improper footwear can contribute to back, hip, and joint pain during pregnancy. Your feet are the foundation of your posture, and when they are not properly supported, it can throw off your entire alignment. Poor foot support can lead to compensatory movements in your knees, hips, and back, causing unnecessary strain on your joints.

The right footwear, particularly shoes with good arch support, can help maintain proper posture and reduce the strain on your joints. This can significantly reduce the likelihood of developing pain in your lower back, hips, and knees as your body accommodates your growing belly.

Stylish Flats, Sneakers, and Sandals for Pregnant Women

When it comes to finding shoes that support pregnancy, style doesn't have to be sacrificed for comfort. There are plenty of stylish options that cater to the unique needs of pregnant women, providing both support and aesthetic appeal. Below are some of the best footwear options for expectant mothers, including flats, sneakers, and sandals that combine functionality with style.

1. Flats: Versatile and Supportive

Flats are a popular choice for pregnant women because they offer a combination of comfort and style without the risks that come with wearing high heels. However, not all flats are created equal, and it's important to choose pairs that provide adequate support and cushioning.

- Ballet Flats with Arch Support: Many ballet flats are designed for fashion rather than comfort, so look for those with built-in arch support and cushioned insoles. Flats that feature padded footbeds and flexible soles help distribute your weight more evenly and reduce pressure on your feet. Some brands now offer orthopedic ballet flats that are both stylish and supportive, perfect for daily wear during pregnancy.

- Loafers and Slip-On Flats: Loafers and slip-on flats are another excellent option for pregnant women. They provide a bit more structure than traditional ballet flats, which can make them more supportive. Look for loafers with a soft, breathable upper and a cushioned sole to keep your feet comfortable. Loafers with elastic panels or adjustable straps can also accommodate any swelling that may occur as your pregnancy progresses.

- Espadrilles and Flat Mules: If you're looking for a more casual option, espadrilles and flat mules are fashionable alternatives. Espadrilles with woven jute soles provide a stylish, summery look while offering a flat base for your feet. Mules, on the other hand, are easy to slip on and off, making them ideal for pregnant women who may struggle with bending over to tie shoes.

2. Sneakers: Maximum Comfort and Support

Sneakers are a must-have for any pregnant woman who is frequently on her feet. They offer excellent cushioning, support, and shock absorption, making them ideal for activities like walking, light exercise, or running errands.

- Cushioned Running Shoes: Running shoes are designed to provide maximum support and shock absorption, making them perfect for pregnant women who need extra comfort. Look for shoes with a breathable mesh upper, plenty of arch support, and a cushioned mid sole. Many brands offer running shoes with memory foam insoles, which conform to the shape of your foot and provide customized comfort.

- Slip-On Sneakers: Slip-on sneakers are a great option for pregnant women who want the comfort of a sneaker without the hassle of laces. These shoes are easy to put on and take off, especially as your belly grows and it becomes more difficult to bend over. Slip-on sneakers offer the same support and cushioning as traditional sneakers, making them ideal for daily wear.

- Orthopedic Sneakers: For women experiencing significant foot pain or discomfort during pregnancy, orthopedic sneakers provide additional support. These shoes are designed to promote proper foot alignment and reduce the risk of developing conditions like plantar fasciitis or flat feet. Many orthopedic sneakers feature a wider toe box to accommodate swelling, as well as contoured footbeds for enhanced arch support.

3. Sandals: Comfortable and Airy for Warmer Weather

During the warmer months, sandals become the go-to option for many pregnant women. The key is to find sandals that offer both style and comfort while providing the necessary support for your changing feet.

- Supportive Flat Sandals: Look for flat sandals with built-in arch support and cushioned footbeds. Brands that specialize in orthopedic sandals often provide options that are stylish but also designed to promote proper alignment and reduce strain on your feet. Sandals with adjustable straps are ideal, as they allow you to loosen the fit if your feet swell throughout the day.

- Slide Sandals: Slide sandals are easy to slip on and off, making them perfect for pregnant women who want a quick, comfortable footwear option. Many slide sandals come with cushioned soles and wide straps, providing both comfort and a secure fit. They can be worn around the house, on casual outings, or at the beach, offering versatility for different activities.

- Wedge Sandals: If you want a bit of height without the discomfort of high heels, wedge sandals are a great alternative. Wedges provide more stability and support than traditional heels, making them safer to wear during pregnancy. Opt for wedge sandals with a lower heel and a cushioned insole to ensure comfort.

Tips for Choosing Maternity-Specific Footwear

Choosing the right footwear during pregnancy requires more than just finding shoes that fit. You need to consider factors such as support, flexibility, breath-ability, and how well the shoes will accommodate your changing body. Here are some tips to help you choose the best maternity-specific footwear:

1. Prioritize Arch Support and Cushioning

As your feet bear the extra weight of pregnancy, proper arch support becomes even more critical. Shoes with good arch support help distribute your weight evenly across your feet, reducing the risk of pain and injury. Cushioned soles, particularly those made from memory foam or gel, provide additional comfort by absorbing the impact of walking and standing.

2. Opt for Adjustable and Flexible Shoes

Pregnancy often comes with swelling in the feet, which can make your usual shoe size uncomfortable. To accommodate this, choose shoes with adjustable straps, elastic panels, or laces that can be loosened or tightened as needed.

Flexible materials like mesh, leather, or stretch fabrics allow your shoes to adapt to any changes in foot size and shape, ensuring you remain comfortable throughout the day.

3. Choose Breathable Materials

Pregnancy hormones can cause your body temperature to rise, leading to hot, sweaty feet. To combat this, opt for shoes made from breathable materials like mesh, cotton, or leather. Breathable shoes help keep your feet cool and dry, reducing the risk of overheating and discomfort, especially during warmer months or long days on your feet. Synthetic materials that don't allow your feet to breathe can lead to excessive sweating and increase the likelihood of developing blisters or foot odor.

4. Avoid High Heels and Unstable Footwear

During pregnancy, wearing high heels or shoes with minimal support can throw off your balance, increasing the risk of falling. As your center of gravity shifts and your joints become looser due to hormonal changes, maintaining stability becomes more challenging. It's best to avoid high heels and opt for lower-heeled shoes, flats, or wedge sandals that provide more support and help you maintain your balance.

- Low-Heeled Shoes: If you prefer a bit of height, choose shoes with low, block heels or wedges. These styles provide more stability than stilettos or narrow heels and help distribute your weight more evenly across your feet.

- Wide-Toe Box: Shoes with a wide-toe box give your feet plenty of room to move and expand, preventing the shoes from feeling too tight or constricting. This is especially important in later pregnancy when swelling is more likely.

5. Consider Orthotic Inserts

If you find that your regular shoes are not providing enough support, orthotic inserts can be a game-changer during pregnancy. Custom orthotic insoles are designed to fit the unique shape of your feet and can provide extra arch support, cushioning, and stability. Many stores offer over-the-counter orthotic inserts that can be easily added to your existing shoes, providing an extra layer of comfort and preventing common foot problems like plantar fasciitis.

6. Try Shoes on Later in the Day

Feet tend to swell as the day goes on, especially during pregnancy. To ensure that your new shoes will fit comfortably even when your feet are slightly swollen, it's a good idea to try them on in the afternoon or evening. This will give you a better sense of how the shoes will feel throughout the day and help you avoid buying footwear that may feel too tight or restrictive after a few hours of wear.

7. Don't Forget About Compression Socks

Compression socks are not technically footwear, but they are an excellent addition to your maternity wardrobe, especially if you're experiencing significant swelling or discomfort in your legs and feet. Compression socks help improve circulation and reduce swelling by applying gentle pressure to your legs and feet. They can be worn with sneakers, flats, or even sandals during pregnancy to promote better blood flow and prevent conditions like varicose veins or deep vein thrombosis (DVT).

Footwear plays a crucial role in ensuring that pregnant women stay comfortable and supported throughout the different stages of pregnancy. As your body changes and your feet experience new challenges like swelling, discomfort, and balance issues, choosing the right shoes can significantly impact your overall well-being.

From stylish ballet flats and slip-on sneakers to supportive sandals and orthopedic shoes, there are numerous options available that combine comfort with fashion. The key is to prioritize shoes that offer ample arch support, cushioning, and flexibility, allowing for the changes your feet will undergo during pregnancy. Additionally, opting for breathable materials, adjustable features, and wide-toe boxes will help you maintain comfort as your body and feet evolve.

By carefully selecting shoes that cater to your specific pregnancy needs, you can prevent foot-related issues like swelling, foot pain, and poor posture, ensuring that you remain active and comfortable throughout your pregnancy journey. Investing in quality, supportive footwear now will not only benefit you during pregnancy but also promote better foot health in the postpartum period, when your body is recovering and adjusting once again.

Ultimately, pregnancy is a time of significant change, and having the right footwear is essential for navigating these changes with ease and comfort. Whether you're walking, exercising, or simply going about your day-to-day activities, the right shoes can make all the difference in how you feel—both physically and emotionally.

Accessorizing Your Maternity Look

ccessorizing during pregnancy offers a wonderful opportunity to enhance your maternity wardrobe, express your personal style, and add versatility to your outfits. Whether you're in the early stages of pregnancy or nearing your due date, the right accessories can transform a basic maternity outfit into something fashionable and chic. While comfort remains a priority during pregnancy, accessories allow you to keep your style fresh without compromising on practicality.

In this chapter, we'll explore how scarves, belts, and jewelry can elevate your maternity style, practical yet stylish handbags and diaper bags that serve as fashion accessories, and other essential items like hats and sunglasses that can enhance your look during outdoor adventures. By the end of this chapter, you'll have a comprehensive guide to accessorizing your maternity wardrobe in a way that combines fashion with functionality.

Scarves, Belts, and Jewelry to Enhance Your Maternity Style

Accessories like scarves, belts, and jewelry can completely change the look of an outfit, giving you endless possibilities to mix and match pieces while adding a touch of personality to your maternity wardrobe. These simple yet effective accessories can help you stay stylish while highlighting your bump or drawing attention to your favorite features.

1. Scarves: Versatile and Stylish

Scarves are a versatile accessory that can be used year-round to add texture, color, and dimension to your maternity outfits. From lightweight, breezy scarves in the summer to cozy, thick scarves in the winter, there's a scarf for every season and occasion. Scarves are particularly useful during pregnancy because they offer coverage, style, and comfort without constricting your growing belly.

- Lightweight Scarves for Warm Weather: In the warmer months, opt for lightweight scarves made from materials like cotton, silk, or linen. These scarves can be draped loosely around your neck or shoulders to add a splash of color to a basic maternity dress or top. They can also be tied into different styles—such as a wrap, shawl, or even a headscarf—for a creative touch.

- Chunky Knit Scarves for Cooler Weather: In colder weather, chunky knit scarves provide warmth and style. Look for oversize scarves or infinity scarves that can be wrapped around your neck multiple times, creating a cozy yet fashionable look. Pair them with maternity sweaters or jackets for an extra layer of warmth and comfort.

- Patterned Scarves to Add Interest: Scarves with bold patterns, such as florals, stripes, or geometric designs, can add visual interest to solid-colored maternity outfits. They serve as a great way to draw attention upward, away from your bump if you prefer a more balanced silhouette. Pair a patterned scarf with a neutral maternity dress or tunic to create a stylish, effortless look.

2. Belts: Defining Your Silhouette

Belts are an incredibly useful accessory during pregnancy because they help define your shape and highlight your bump in a flattering way. Whether you're in your first trimester or third, belts can accentuate your waistline and add a polished finish to your maternity outfit. Additionally, belts can be used to transition your pre-pregnancy clothes into your maternity wardrobe by cinching loose tops or dresses at the empire waist.

- Empire Waist Belts: During pregnancy, empire waist belts—worn just below the bust—are a great way to draw attention to the slimmest part of your body while showcasing your growing bump. Wide belts in soft materials work particularly well for defining the empire waist without causing discomfort. Pair an empire waist belt with a flowy maternity dress to create a flattering, elegant silhouette.

- Adjustable Belts for Flexibility: Adjustable belts, such as those with buckles or ties, are ideal for pregnancy because they can grow with you as your belly expands. These belts allow you to customize the fit and ensure that you're comfortable throughout your pregnancy. Soft, elastic belts are also great options for offering flexibility while still maintaining a stylish look.

- Statement Belts for Added Flair: If you're looking to make a statement, consider a bold belt with decorative elements like studs, beading, or embellishments. Statement belts can add flair to a simple maternity dress or tunic and make your outfit stand out for special occasions. Just make sure the belt is comfortable and not too tight around your growing belly.

3. Jewelry: Adding Personality and Elegance

Jewelry is an easy way to express your personal style and elevate your maternity look, whether you're dressing up for a formal event or keeping it casual for a day out. From dainty necklaces to bold statement earrings, jewelry adds the finishing touch to any outfit and helps draw attention to your favorite features.

- Long Necklaces to Complement Your Bump: Long necklaces are perfect for elongating your torso and drawing attention to your baby bump. Opt for necklaces with pendants or layered designs that fall just above or below your belly. These necklaces can add a touch of elegance to a basic maternity dress and help balance your silhouette.

- Statement Earrings for Special Occasions: Statement earrings are an excellent choice for adding a bold pop of color or sparkle to your maternity outfits, especially for special events. Whether you prefer chandelier earrings, oversize hoops, or intricate drop earrings, these pieces can enhance your look without overwhelming your overall style.

- Bracelets and Bangles: Bracelets and bangles are a great way to accessorize your maternity wardrobe while keeping it light and comfortable. Layering multiple bangles or wearing a single statement cuff can add a chic element to your outfit. Bracelets with adjustable clasps or stretchy bands are ideal during pregnancy to accommodate any swelling in your wrists.

Practical Handbags and Diaper Bags that Double as Fashion Accessories

As your pregnancy progresses, practical accessories become even more important. A well-chosen handbag or diaper bag can serve both functional and aesthetic purposes, allowing you to carry all your essentials while still looking stylish. When choosing a maternity-friendly handbag or diaper bag, look for options that offer plenty of storage, easy access, and comfort without sacrificing fashion.

1. Cross body Bags: Stylish and Functional

Cross body bags are a great option for pregnant women because they distribute weight evenly across your body, helping to prevent back and shoulder strain. These bags are typically smaller and lighter than traditional handbags, making them ideal for carrying just the essentials, such as your phone, wallet, and keys. Cross body bags come in a variety of styles, from casual to more formal, so you can choose one that complements your outfit while keeping you hands-free.

- Adjustable Straps for Comfort: Look for cross body bags with adjustable straps that allow you to customize the length and ensure a comfortable fit as your body changes. Soft, padded straps can also help prevent the bag from digging into your shoulder.

- Compact but Spacious: While cross body bags are generally smaller, opt for one with multiple compartments or pockets to help keep your belongings organized. This makes it easier to access your essentials without rummaging through a large bag.

2. Tote Bags: Roomy and Versatile

Tote bags are a popular choice for pregnant women because they offer ample storage space for all your daily essentials. Whether you're heading to work, running errands, or preparing for a day out, a tote bag provides the space you need to carry everything from water bottles and snacks to maternity documents and even a spare outfit.

- Lightweight and Durable: When choosing a tote bag, look for lightweight materials that won't add unnecessary weight. Leather, canvas, or nylon totes are durable options that provide both fashion and function. Avoid heavy or overly structured bags that could become cumbersome as your belly grows.

- Multiple Compartments for Organization: A tote bag with multiple compartments is essential for keeping your items organized and easily accessible. Look for bags with zippered pockets, side pockets, or internal dividers to help keep everything in its place.

3. Diaper Bags as Fashion Accessories

Once your baby arrives, a diaper bag will become one of your most important accessories. Fortunately, modern diaper bags are designed to be both practical and stylish, allowing you to carry all your baby essentials without sacrificing your fashion sense. Many diaper bags now resemble trendy handbags or backpacks, offering plenty of storage space while complementing your everyday look.

- Convertible Diaper Bags: Convertible diaper bags can be worn as a backpack, shoulder bag, or cross body bag, offering versatility and comfort. These bags are ideal for busy moms who need to be hands-free while still carrying all their baby gear. Look for bags with padded straps, durable materials, and plenty of pockets for easy organization.

- Chic, Minimalist Designs: Diaper bags no longer have to scream "baby gear." Many brands offer chic, minimalist designs that look like stylish handbags or designer totes. These bags feature all the functionality of a traditional diaper bag, such as insulated bottle holders and wipe-able changing mats, while still maintaining a sleek, fashionable appearance.

- Neutral Colors for Versatility: Neutral-colored diaper bags in shades like black, tan, or gray can easily be paired with any outfit, making them a versatile accessory for both moms and dads. These bags can seamlessly transition from baby duty to a stylish day out without looking out of place.

Hats, Sunglasses, and Other Accessories for Outdoor Adventures

During pregnancy, it's important to protect yourself from the elements, especially when spending time outdoors. Whether you're enjoying a sunny day at the park, taking a relaxing walk, or heading to the beach, the right accessories can help you stay comfortable and stylish while ensuring that you're protected from the sun, wind, or rain.

1. Hats: Fashionable and Functional

Hats are a must-have accessory for pregnant women who spend time outdoors, offering both sun protection and a stylish addition to any outfit. Whether you're looking for a casual, everyday hat or something more elegant for a special occasion, there are plenty of options to choose from.

Wide-Brimmed Hats: Wide-brimmed hats provide excellent sun protection, shielding your face, neck, and shoulders from harmful UV rays. They are a stylish and functional option for outdoor adventures, whether you're heading to the beach, a park, or a garden party. Look for hats made from lightweight, breathable materials like straw or cotton to keep you cool and comfortable.

- Fedoras and Sun Hats: Fedoras offer a slightly more structured and fashionable look while still providing sun protection. They pair well with casual maternity outfits like maxi dresses, jeans, or tunics. Sun hats, on the other hand, are more relaxed and great for beach outings, walks, or casual outdoor gatherings. Both styles can be dressed up or down, depending on your look.

- Caps for Casual Outings: If you're looking for a more casual, everyday hat, a baseball cap or a trucker hat is a great option. These hats are perfect for outdoor exercise, errands, or relaxed weekend activities. They help protect your face from the sun while keeping you cool and comfortable.

2. Sunglasses: Essential for Eye Protection and Style

Sunglasses are an essential accessory for pregnant women spending time outdoors. Not only do they protect your eyes from harmful UV rays, but they also add a fashionable touch to any outfit. Pregnancy hormones can make your skin and eyes more sensitive to sunlight, so wearing sunglasses is crucial for comfort and safety.

- Over-sized Sunglasses for a Glamorous Look: Over-sized sunglasses offer extra coverage and a touch of Hollywood glamour. They protect a larger portion of your face from the sun while adding an effortlessly chic element to your outfit. Whether you're lounging by the pool or attending an outdoor brunch, oversize sunglasses are a perfect way to elevate your maternity look.

- Classic Aviators or Wayfarers: If you prefer a more classic, timeless style, aviators or wayfarer sunglasses are great options. These sunglasses are versatile and can be worn with casual or dressy maternity outfits. Aviators offer a sleek, modern look, while wayfarers are more retro-inspired, making them a stylish choice for various occasions.

- Polarized Sunglasses for Extra Protection: When spending extended time outdoors, polarized sunglasses provide extra protection by reducing glare from surfaces like water, sand, or pavement. These are particularly useful for beach trips, hiking, or outdoor exercise. Polarized lenses help reduce eye strain and improve clarity, making them a practical and stylish choice for active moms-to-be.

3. Other Outdoor Accessories

When preparing for outdoor adventures, especially during pregnancy, a few additional accessories can help enhance your comfort while keeping you stylish.

- Lightweight Scarves and Shawls: A lightweight scarf or shawl can offer extra protection from the sun or a light breeze. Choose scarves made from natural, breathable fabrics like cotton, silk, or linen. These accessories can be draped over your shoulders, wrapped around your neck, or used as a cover-up at the beach.

- Umbrellas for Shade and Rain Protection: Whether you're shielding yourself from the sun or staying dry in the rain, a stylish umbrella can come in handy during outdoor outings. Look for compact umbrellas that can easily fit into your handbag, ensuring you're always prepared for unpredictable weather.

- Water Bottles: Staying hydrated is crucial during pregnancy, especially when you're spending time outdoors. A chic, reusable water bottle is a practical accessory that can also serve as a fashion statement. Choose a bottle in a color or pattern that complements your style, and make sure it's easy to carry with you on outdoor adventures.

Accessorizing during pregnancy is all about finding the right balance between style and comfort. Whether you're dressing for a casual day out, attending a formal event, or preparing for an outdoor adventure, the right accessories can enhance your maternity wardrobe and allow you to express your personal style.

Scarves, belts, and jewelry offer a simple way to elevate any maternity outfit, while practical handbags and diaper bags provide both function and fashion. Hats and sunglasses protect you from the elements while adding a stylish touch to your look. Ultimately, the key to accessorizing during pregnancy is to choose pieces that make you feel confident, comfortable, and ready for whatever your day brings.

By thoughtfully selecting accessories that complement your outfits and cater to your specific needs, you can maintain your sense of style throughout your pregnancy and beyond. Whether you're enjoying a relaxing day at home, preparing for a special occasion, or heading out for an outdoor adventure, these accessories will help you look and feel your best at every stage of your maternity journey.

Affordable Maternity Fashion on a Budget

Pregnancy is a unique time in life, and for many women, it requires adjusting their wardrobe to accommodate their changing bodies. However, maternity fashion doesn't have to be expensive. With the right strategies, it's possible to find stylish, comfortable maternity clothes without breaking the bank. Whether you're looking for budget-friendly retail options, want to explore secondhand and thrift stores, or simply want to be more resourceful with your wardrobe, there are plenty of ways to look great throughout your pregnancy while sticking to a budget.

This chapter will guide you through finding affordable maternity clothes, introduce the best places to shop both online and in-store, and offer tips for navigating secondhand and thrift shopping. By the end, you'll have all the tools you need to build a stylish maternity wardrobe without overspending.

Finding Stylish Maternity Clothes Without Breaking the Bank

One of the main challenges during pregnancy is finding clothes that fit well and make you feel confident without spending a fortune. Because your body changes throughout each trimester, buying an entirely new wardrobe can seem daunting and expensive. However, with a bit of planning and smart shopping, you can create a versatile, functional maternity wardrobe at an affordable price.

1. Prioritize Versatile Basics

When building a maternity wardrobe on a budget, the key is to focus on versatile basics that can be mixed and matched to create multiple outfits. Instead of splurging on trendy, one-time pieces, invest in timeless basics that will work for a variety of occasions.

- Maternity Leggings: One of the most versatile pieces for any pregnant woman is a good pair of maternity leggings. They are comfortable, stretchy, and can be paired with different tops and tunics for both casual and dressier looks. Leggings can be worn throughout pregnancy and even post-pregnancy.

- Basic Maternity Dresses: A simple, solid-colored maternity dress can go a long way. Choose dresses in neutral shades like black, gray, or navy, which can be dressed up with accessories or layered with different jackets or cardigans. Stretchy, body-hugging dresses with ruching along the sides will grow with your belly and maintain a flattering shape.

- Maternity Tops and T-Shirts: Invest in a few maternity tops and t-shirts that can be mixed with jeans, skirts, or leggings. Tops with side ruching or empire waists provide a comfortable fit as your belly grows. Choose tops in neutral colors and basic patterns that can be paired with different bottoms.

- Maternity Jeans: A pair of affordable maternity jeans is a must-have for a casual wardrobe. Look for jeans with elastic waistbands or over-the-belly panels that provide both comfort and support. They can be paired with various tops for casual outings or dressed up with blouses for a more polished look.

2. Maximize the Use of Non-Maternity Clothing

You don't need to completely overhaul your wardrobe during pregnancy— many non-maternity clothes can still work for your changing body. The key is to look for loose-fitting or stretchy items in your existing wardrobe or purchase non-maternity pieces that can accommodate your bump.

- Stretchy Maxi Dresses and Tunics: Maxi dresses and tunics, particularly those made from stretchy fabrics, can accommodate a growing belly. These loose, flowy pieces provide plenty of room for movement and are stylish for both casual and formal occasions.

- Empire Waist Dresses: Dresses with an empire waist (which cinches just below the bust and flares out) are often perfect for pregnancy. They provide room for your bump while still giving you a flattering shape. Look for empire waist dresses in your existing wardrobe or consider purchasing non-maternity versions that will work during and after pregnancy.

- Over-sized Sweaters and Cardigans: Over-sized sweaters and cardigans are perfect for layering over maternity tops and dresses. These non-maternity pieces offer warmth and comfort while adding versatility to your wardrobe.

- Adjustable Waist Skirts and Pants: Many skirts and pants have adjustable waistbands or drawstrings that can be loosened as your belly grows. These are great budget-friendly options for those who want to wear non-maternity clothing throughout their pregnancy.

3. Take Advantage of Sales and Discounts

One of the easiest ways to save money on maternity clothes is to keep an eye out for sales, promotions, and discounts. Many maternity brands offer seasonal sales or discount codes, and you can often find great deals by shopping during holiday promotions.

- Sign Up for Newsletters: Many online stores offer exclusive discounts to customers who sign up for their newsletters. Take advantage of this by subscribing to your favorite maternity brands or retailers and waiting for discounts to roll in. Many stores also offer welcome discounts, giving you a percentage off your first purchase.

- End-of-Season Sales: Shopping during end-of-season sales is a great way to find discounted maternity wear. These sales often offer deep discounts on items that retailers are trying to clear out to make room for new inventory. You can stock up on off-season items like sweaters, jackets, or summer dresses at a fraction of the original price.

- Shop Off-Price Retailers: Off-price retailers like T.J. Maxx, Ross, and Marshalls often carry maternity clothes at significantly lower prices than traditional retail stores. You may need to search through the racks, but it's possible to find high-quality maternity pieces at a discount.

Best Places to Shop for Affordable Maternity Clothes (Online and In-Store)

There are many places, both online and in physical stores, where you can find affordable maternity clothing. From fast-fashion retailers to specialty maternity stores, shopping around and comparing prices can help you stay within your budget. Here are some of the best places to shop for budget-friendly maternity wear:

1. Online Retailers

Online shopping offers convenience and often provides access to a wider range of maternity options than brick-and-mortar stores. Many online retailers specialize in affordable, trendy maternity wear, making it easy to find stylish pieces without spending too much.

- ASOS: ASOS is known for its trendy, affordable fashion, and its maternity section is no exception. ASOS offers a wide variety of maternity dresses, tops, jeans, and active-wear at reasonable prices. The retailer often runs sales and promotions, so it's a great place to find budget-friendly maternity clothes.

- H&M: H&M's maternity section offers stylish and affordable basics like maternity leggings, dresses, and nursing tops. H&M is known for offering a balance of trendy and classic pieces, making it a go-to retailer for budget-conscious shoppers. Their sales section often features deeply discounted maternity items.

- Old Navy: Old Navy's maternity line is perfect for moms-to-be on a budget. The brand offers affordable maternity jeans, tops, active-wear, and dresses. With frequent sales and promotions, Old Navy is a great place to stock up on comfortable, casual maternity pieces.

- Amazon: Amazon offers an extensive range of maternity clothes from various brands at affordable prices. Whether you're looking for basics like maternity leggings or more specialized items like nursing tops or dresses, Amazon's competitive pricing and Prime shipping options make it a convenient option for maternity shopping.

2. In-Store Retailers

For those who prefer to shop in person, many stores carry maternity lines at reasonable prices. In-store shopping allows you to try on items to ensure they fit well, which is especially important during pregnancy when your body is constantly changing.

- Target: Target's maternity section, known as the Isabel Maternity line, offers a great selection of affordable, comfortable maternity clothes. From everyday basics like leggings and tees to stylish dresses, Target provides budget-friendly options for expectant moms.

- Walmart: Walmart's maternity section offers affordable maternity basics like leggings, jeans, and tops. While the selection may not be as extensive as some other retailers, Walmart provides low-cost options for women who need to expand their maternity wardrobe on a tight budget.

- Kohl's: Kohl's carries an affordable line of maternity clothes, including basics, work-wear, and casual pieces. The store frequently offers sales, promotions, and Kohl's Cash, making it a budget-friendly option for maternity shopping.

- Gap: Gap's maternity line is known for its stylish yet comfortable pieces that cater to moms-to-be who want quality clothes at affordable prices. With frequent sales and promotions, Gap is a great place to find maternity jeans, dresses, and casual wear.

3. Maternity Subscription Boxes

If you're unsure where to start with maternity fashion or don't have time to shop, maternity subscription boxes can offer a convenient and budget-friendly solution. These services deliver curated maternity clothes to your doorstep, often at discounted prices.

- Stitch Fix Maternity: Stitch Fix offers a maternity styling service where a personal stylist curates a selection of maternity clothes based on your preferences and needs. You pay a styling fee, which is credited toward any items you choose to keep. The flexibility to try on clothes at home before purchasing makes this a convenient option for busy moms-to-be.

- Le Tote Maternity: Le Tote is a clothing rental service that offers a maternity-specific subscription box. You can rent maternity clothes and exchange them as often as you like, making it an affordable way to wear trendy maternity fashion without committing to permanent purchases.

Tips for Secondhand and Thrift Shopping for Maternity Wear

Secondhand and thrift shopping are excellent ways to save money on maternity clothes, especially considering that maternity clothes are often worn for a limited time. By shopping secondhand, you can find high-quality, gently used maternity pieces at a fraction of the cost of buying new.

1. Thrift Stores and Consignment Shops

Thrift stores and consignment shops are treasure troves for finding affordable maternity wear. Many women donate or consign their maternity clothes after giving birth, leaving behind stylish, gently used pieces that are perfect for expectant mothers looking to save money. Shopping at thrift stores or consignment shops not only helps you stick to a budget but also allows you to find unique and high-quality items that you might not see elsewhere. Here are some tips for finding great secondhand maternity wear:

1.1 Check Local Thrift Stores Regularly

Because maternity clothes are often only worn for a few months, they tend to be in good condition when donated to thrift stores. Visit your local thrift stores frequently, as their inventory changes often. Be patient and persistent, and you're likely to find great deals on maternity wear. Some larger thrift chains, like Goodwill or Salvation Army, may have dedicated maternity sections, making it easier to browse.

- Be Open-Minded: While you might not always find a specific item you're looking for, be open to different styles and brands. Thrift shopping can sometimes yield unexpected treasures, and you might discover pieces that you wouldn't have considered if shopping new.

- Look for Quality Fabrics: When shopping secondhand, focus on items made from durable, high-quality fabrics like cotton, spandex, or jersey. These materials tend to hold up well over time and are more likely to be in good condition even after a previous owner has worn them. Check for any signs of wear, such as stretching or fading, especially around seams and hems.

1.2 Consignment Stores for Gently Used Maternity Wear

Consignment stores often carry gently used or like-new maternity clothes from well-known brands. These stores curate their inventory more carefully than regular thrift stores, so you're more likely to find high-quality maternity pieces. Some consignment shops specialize in maternity and baby clothes, making them ideal places to find everything you need for your pregnancy wardrobe at a fraction of the cost.

- Maternity-Specific Consignment Stores: Look for consignment stores in your area that specialize in maternity or children's clothing. These stores are typically more selective about the condition of the items they accept, so you can often find high-quality maternity wear at significantly lower prices than retail.

- Bundle Discounts: Many consignment shops offer discounts when you buy multiple items or bundle clothing together. Take advantage of these deals to stock up on essentials like maternity jeans, leggings, and tops.

2. Online Secondhand Shopping

In addition to local thrift and consignment stores, there are numerous online platforms where you can buy and sell secondhand maternity clothes. These platforms offer a convenient way to shop for affordable maternity wear from the comfort of your home, and they often have a wide selection of sizes, styles, and brands.

- ThredUP: ThredUP is one of the largest online consignment stores and offers a dedicated maternity section. You can find high-quality, gently used maternity clothes at discounted prices, including popular brands like Gap, Old Navy, and Motherhood Maternity. ThredUP also allows you to filter by size, brand, and price range, making it easy to find exactly what you're looking for.

- Posh mark: Posh mark is another popular platform where individuals sell their secondhand clothing, including maternity wear. Sellers list their items with photos and descriptions, and you can negotiate prices or bundle items to get discounts. Posh mark offers a range of maternity brands, from affordable fast-fashion to designer labels.

- Facebook Marketplace and Buy-Sell Groups: Facebook Marketplace and local buy-sell groups are excellent resources for finding secondhand maternity clothes at low prices. These platforms allow you to search for items in your area and arrange pick-up or delivery with the seller. Joining local mom groups or maternity-specific buy-sell groups can also help you find great deals on gently used maternity wear.

3. Rent Maternity Clothes

If you don't want to invest in an entire maternity wardrobe but still want access to stylish, high-quality clothes, consider renting maternity wear. Renting allows you to wear designer or trendier items without committing to purchasing them. This option is especially useful for special occasions, such as weddings or baby showers, when you want to wear something elegant but don't want to spend a lot on an item you'll only wear once or twice.

- Rent the Runway: Rent the Runway offers a maternity section where you can rent designer dresses, outfits, and accessories for a fraction of the retail price. Whether you need a dress for a formal event or just want a few trendy pieces to wear during pregnancy, Rent the Runway allows you to wear high-end maternity fashion without the high cost.

- Le Tote: Le Tote, as mentioned earlier, offers a maternity subscription box where you can rent clothes and exchange them as often as you like. This service is perfect for moms-to-be who want to refresh their maternity wardrobe regularly without making a long-term financial commitment to new clothes.

4. DIY and Up-cycling Tips for Budget-Friendly Maternity Wear

If you're feeling creative and want to make the most of your existing wardrobe, there are several DIY and up-cycling techniques you can use to adapt your pre-pregnancy clothes into maternity wear. These budget-friendly solutions allow you to re-purpose what you already own, reducing the need to buy new items.

- DIY Belly Bands: A belly band is a stretchy piece of fabric that wraps around your waist, allowing you to wear your regular jeans or pants unbuttoned. If you don't want to buy a new belly band, you can easily make one using a stretchy, elastic material or even by cutting off the waistband of an old pair of leggings. The belly band holds your pants in place while providing coverage for your growing bump.

- Turn Dresses into Maternity Wear: Non-maternity dresses that are loose-fitting, stretchy, or empire-waist can be adapted into maternity wear. You can add a belt above your bump to accentuate your waist or layer the dress with maternity leggings for added comfort.

- Transform Tops into Nursing-Friendly Clothes: Many maternity tops and dresses can be turned into nursing-friendly clothes by adding discreet zippers or snaps at the bust. This allows you to continue wearing the same clothes post-pregnancy while making them functional for breastfeeding.

Building a stylish, comfortable maternity wardrobe doesn't have to be expensive. With a few smart shopping strategies, it's possible to find budget-friendly maternity wear that suits your lifestyle and evolving body. Whether you're shopping for new clothes online or in-store, exploring secondhand and thrift options, or even renting pieces for special occasions, there are plenty of ways to stay fashionable without overspending.

By prioritizing versatile basics, mixing non-maternity clothes with your new maternity pieces, and taking advantage of sales and secondhand shopping platforms, you can create a wardrobe that's both practical and stylish. Remember that pregnancy is a temporary phase, so focus on finding pieces that will work for the duration of your pregnancy while allowing you to stay within your budget.

Ultimately, with the right approach, you can look and feel great throughout your pregnancy without the need to break the bank. Whether you're heading to work, attending a social event, or simply lounging at home, your maternity wardrobe can be both functional and fashionable with a little creativity and resourcefulness.

DIY and Up-cycling: Maternity Fashion Hacks

Pregnancy can be a time of both joy and challenge when it comes to dressing your ever-changing body. As your bump grows, your regular clothes may start to feel tight or uncomfortable. But instead of purchasing an entirely new wardrobe, there are plenty of DIY and up-cycling hacks that can help you re-purpose your pre-pregnancy clothes, extend the life of your maternity wardrobe, and even transform old maternity wear into stylish post-pregnancy outfits.

In this chapter, we'll explore creative and practical ways to adapt your existing wardrobe for pregnancy. You'll learn how to make easy DIY alterations to your pre-pregnancy clothes, discover hacks that will help you expand your maternity wardrobe without spending a fortune, and find out how to up-cycle old maternity clothes into fashionable, functional items for post-pregnancy use. By the end of this chapter, you'll have all the tools you need to create a versatile and sustainable wardrobe that works before, during, and after pregnancy.

How to Re-purpose Your Pre-Pregnancy Clothes for Maternity Use

One of the best ways to save money during pregnancy is to re-purpose the clothes you already own. While some items in your pre-pregnancy wardrobe may no longer fit comfortably, many pieces can be adjusted or worn differently to accommodate your growing bump. With a little creativity, you can avoid purchasing expensive maternity clothes and make the most of what you have.

1. Stretchy and Loose-Fitting Clothes

The easiest pre-pregnancy clothes to re-purpose during pregnancy are those that are already stretchy or loose-fitting. These items naturally accommodate a growing belly and provide the comfort you need without any alterations.

- Maxi Dresses and Skirts: Maxi dresses and skirts are a great option during pregnancy because they provide plenty of room for your bump while still looking stylish. Stretchy fabrics like jersey or cotton blends are particularly comfortable, and many non-maternity maxi dresses can be worn throughout pregnancy without any adjustments. Pair them with a belt above your bump to create a flattering silhouette.

- Empire Waist Dresses and Tops: Empire waist dresses and tops, which cinch just below the bust and flow out over the belly, are perfect for pregnancy. These pieces are already designed to accommodate a fuller figure, making them ideal for re-purposing as maternity wear. If you have empire waist dresses or tops in your pre-pregnancy wardrobe, you can continue wearing them without needing any alterations.

- Tunic Tops: Loose-fitting tunic tops are another versatile item that can be worn during pregnancy. Tunics provide extra length and coverage, making them perfect for pairing with maternity leggings or jeans. If you have tunics made from stretchy or breathable fabrics, you'll find them especially comfortable as your bump grows.

2. Re-purposing Pants and Jeans with a Belly Band

One of the most common challenges during pregnancy is finding pants and jeans that fit comfortably as your belly expands. Instead of buying new maternity pants right away, you can use a belly band to extend the life of your pre-pregnancy bottoms. A belly band is a stretchy fabric band that wraps around your waist and covers the top of your unbuttoned pants, allowing you to wear your regular jeans or trousers without needing to fasten them.

- DIY Belly Band: If you don't want to purchase a belly band, you can easily make your own. Simply take an old, stretchy tank top or camisole and cut off the bottom portion (from just below the bust). You can wear this makeshift band over the top of your pants to hold them in place while leaving them unbuttoned.

- Hair Tie Trick: Another quick hack to extend the life of your pre-pregnancy pants is the hair tie trick. Loop a hair tie or rubber band through the buttonhole of your pants and then hook it around the button. This gives you a few extra inches of waistband room without needing to buy maternity pants right away.

3. Layering Non-Maternity Clothes

Layering is a great way to make your pre-pregnancy clothes work during pregnancy. By layering stretchy or loose-fitting items with longer cardigans, open-front jackets, or scarves, you can create stylish outfits that provide coverage and comfort.

- Open-Front Cardigans and Blazers: Many cardigans, blazers, and jackets can be worn open during pregnancy, allowing your bump to grow while still giving you a polished, layered look. Pair an open-front cardigan with a basic maternity top and leggings for a comfortable yet put-together outfit.

- Button-Up Shirts as Layers: Button-up shirts may no longer fasten over your growing belly, but they can still be worn open as layering pieces. Wear an unbuttoned shirt over a maternity tank top or stretchy dress for a casual, stylish look. Tie the ends of the shirt just above your bump for a more fitted appearance.

Easy DIY Alterations and Hacks to Expand Your Maternity Wardrobe

If you're handy with a needle and thread (or have access to a sewing machine), there are plenty of simple DIY alterations you can make to your pre-pregnancy clothes to turn them into maternity-friendly garments. These alterations can save you money and allow you to continue wearing your favorite pieces throughout your pregnancy.

1. Adding Side Panels to Tops and Dresses

One of the easiest DIY alterations you can make to your pre-pregnancy tops and dresses is adding side panels. By inserting stretchy fabric panels along the side seams, you can create extra room for your growing belly while keeping the original style of the garment intact.

- How to Add Side Panels: To add side panels, start by cutting open the side seams of the garment. Then, cut two panels of stretchy fabric (such as spandex or jersey) in a triangular shape. Sew the panels into the open side seams, starting at the underarm and tapering down to the hemline. This alteration will give your top or dress the extra width it needs to accommodate your bump.

2. Turning Regular Pants into Maternity Pants

Another popular maternity hack is turning your regular pants into maternity pants by adding an elastic waistband or belly panel. This simple alteration allows you to keep wearing your favorite jeans or trousers without worrying about them becoming too tight as your belly grows.

- How to Add a Belly Panel: Start by cutting off the waistband of your pants. Next, take a stretchy piece of fabric (such as an old t-shirt or stretchy tank top) and sew it to the top of the pants, creating a soft, elastic belly panel. The panel should be long enough to cover your entire belly and provide support as it grows. This hack turns your regular pants into comfortable, maternity-friendly bottoms.

- Elastic Waistband Hack: If you don't want to add a full belly panel, you can simply replace the waistband of your pants with an elastic band. Cut off the waistband of your pants, then sew an elastic band in its place, making sure the elastic is wide enough to stretch comfortably around your belly.

3. Creating Nursing-Friendly Clothes

If you want to plan ahead for the postpartum period, you can make simple DIY alterations to your maternity clothes to turn them into nursing-friendly garments. By adding discreet zippers, snaps, or buttons to tops and dresses, you can make it easier to nurse your baby while still wearing the clothes you love.

- Adding Zippers for Easy Nursing Access: To add zippers to a top or dress, start by cutting small slits along the bust line or side seams. Sew invisible zippers into the slits, making sure they are positioned for easy access during nursing. This alteration allows you to open the zippers when it's time to nurse, then close them for a seamless look.

- Snap Closures for Nursing: Snap closures are another easy way to make a garment nursing-friendly. Simply sew small snaps along the neckline or bust line of a top or dress, allowing you to open and close the garment for nursing without the need for zippers or buttons.

Up-cycling Old Maternity Clothes for Post-Pregnancy Use

Once your pregnancy is over, you may find yourself with a closet full of maternity clothes that no longer fit or suit your needs. Instead of letting these items go to waste, you can up-cycle your old maternity clothes into new, stylish pieces for your postpartum wardrobe or even for everyday wear.

1. Turning Maternity Tops into Nursing Tops

Many maternity tops can be easily up-cycled into nursing tops with a few simple alterations. By adding nursing-friendly features such as zippers, buttons, or wrap fronts, you can continue to wear your favorite maternity tops while nursing your baby.

- Wrap-Style Alteration: One easy way to up-cycle a maternity top into a nursing top is to create a wrap-style front. Cut the front of the top down the middle, then overlap the two sides and sew them in place to create a wrap front. This alteration allows you to easily pull aside the fabric for nursing while still keeping the top stylish and functional.

2. Re-purposing Maternity Dresses into Everyday Wear

Maternity dresses are often designed with extra fabric to accommodate a growing belly, but that doesn't mean they have to be retired after pregnancy. With a few simple adjustments, you can turn your old maternity dresses into stylish everyday wear.

- Shortening a Maxi Dress: If you have a maternity maxi dress that feels too bulky after pregnancy, consider shortening it to knee-length or above-the-knee for a more streamlined look. Simply hem the dress to your desired length, and you'll have a new, flattering piece for your post-pregnancy wardrobe.

- Adding a Belt to Redefine the Waistline: Many maternity dresses have an empire waist that sits just below the bust. After pregnancy, you can redefine the waistline by adding a belt or sash at your natural waistline. This simple adjustment can instantly transform the look of the dress, making it more suitable for your postpartum body. A belt helps create a flattering silhouette and draws attention to your waist, which can be especially helpful as your body gradually returns to its pre-pregnancy shape.

3. Turning Maternity Jeans into Postpartum Jeans

Maternity jeans are designed to be comfortable and stretchy, often with a built-in belly panel or elastic waistband. After pregnancy, you can still wear your maternity jeans by making minor adjustments to the fit, or you can up-cycle them into a new pair of jeans that will suit your postpartum body.

- Removing the Belly Panel: If your maternity jeans have a belly panel, you can remove it and replace it with a regular waistband or elastic waistband. This alteration turns your maternity jeans into a more versatile pair of jeans that can be worn beyond pregnancy. Simply unpick the belly panel from the jeans, and sew a stretchy waistband or even an old waistband from another pair of jeans in its place.

- Turning Maternity Jeans into Shorts: If you no longer need your maternity jeans but want to re-purpose them, consider turning them into shorts for casual, everyday wear. Cut the jeans to your desired length, then hem the edges for a clean finish. This simple alteration allows you to continue wearing your favorite maternity jeans in a new way.

4. Up-cycling Maternity Tops into Lounge-wear or Pajamas

Maternity tops are often made from soft, comfortable fabrics, making them perfect for up-cycling into Lounge-wear or pajamas. Instead of donating or discarding your old maternity tops, consider turning them into cozy, relaxing pieces that you can wear around the house or to bed.

- Turning Maternity Tops into Pajama Tops: If you have maternity tops made from jersey, cotton, or other stretchy fabrics, you can easily convert them into pajama tops. Simply pair them with a pair of soft shorts or lounge pants, and you have a comfortable, easy-to-wear pajama set.

- Making Lounge Shorts or Pants: If you have extra fabric from old maternity dresses or tops, you can use it to make simple lounge shorts or pants. This is a great way to re-purpose fabric that would otherwise go to waste and create comfortable Lounge-wear for your postpartum recovery.

5. Creating New Items from Old Maternity Clothes

Sometimes, old maternity clothes can be up-cycled into completely new items that serve different purposes. If you're feeling creative, consider transforming your maternity garments into useful or fashionable items that can be worn or used in new ways.

- Maternity Dresses to Baby Blankets: If you have a maternity dress made from soft fabric, consider turning it into a baby blanket. Cut the fabric into a large rectangle or square, hem the edges, and you have a cozy, handmade blanket for your little one.

- Tops to Baby Bibs or Burp Cloths: Old maternity tops can be up-cycled into baby bibs or burp cloths. Cut the fabric into the desired shapes, sew along the edges, and add Velcro or snap closures for bibs. This is an easy way to re-purpose fabric while creating useful items for your baby.

- Turning Maternity Clothes into Accessories: If you have old maternity clothes with pretty patterns or colors, consider turning them into accessories like headbands, scarves, or even tote bags. Cut the fabric into strips or squares and sew them into your desired accessory. This is a fun and creative way to keep a piece of your maternity wardrobe while giving it a new life.

Building a maternity wardrobe doesn't have to mean starting from scratch or breaking the bank. With a little creativity and some simple DIY skills, you can re-purpose your pre-pregnancy clothes, make easy alterations to expand your maternity wardrobe, and up-cycle your old maternity wear into stylish, practical pieces for postpartum life. Whether you're using belly bands to extend the life of your jeans or turning old maternity dresses into new garments, these DIY and up-cycling hacks help you get the most out of your wardrobe while saving money.

By re-purposing and up-cycling your clothes, you can create a sustainable and versatile wardrobe that works not only during pregnancy but also after your baby arrives. With the right approach, you can maintain your personal style, stay comfortable, and feel confident without needing to invest in a whole new collection of maternity clothing. From DIY alterations to creative up-cycling projects, the possibilities for transforming your wardrobe are endless, allowing you to embrace your pregnancy journey with both practicality and style.

Body Positivist and Confidence During Pregnancy

Pregnancy is a trans-formative journey that brings about many physical, emotional, and mental changes. While the joy of growing new life is unparalleled, the rapid changes to a pregnant woman's body can sometimes lead to insecurities and struggles with body image. For many women, the experience of watching their bodies expand and change can be challenging, especially in a society that places such a high value on appearance and often promotes unrealistic beauty standards. However, embracing these changes with pride and finding ways to boost self-confidence can lead to a more joyful and empowered pregnancy experience.

In this chapter, we will explore how to cultivate body positivist and confidence during pregnancy by learning to embrace your body's changes, how maternity fashion can be a tool to enhance self-esteem, and ways to address and overcome body image issues that may arise. With the right mindset and self-care strategies, you can develop a stronger connection to your body and a sense of pride in its remarkable abilities.

Embracing Your Body's Changes with Pride

During pregnancy, your body undergoes an incredible transformation to support the development of your baby. These changes, while natural and necessary, can sometimes leave women feeling disconnected from their sense of self or appearance. It's important to recognize that pregnancy is a unique time in life and that your body's changes are a testament to its strength and ability to nurture new life.

1. Shifting Your Perspective on Weight Gain

One of the most noticeable changes during pregnancy is weight gain, which is an essential part of a healthy pregnancy. However, for women who may have struggled with body image in the past or who have internalized societal pressures around thinness, this can be a source of anxiety. It's important to shift your perspective on weight gain by recognizing it as a positive and necessary aspect of growing a baby.

- Focus on Functionality: Instead of viewing weight gain as something negative, focus on the functionality of your body. Your body is gaining weight to provide nourishment for your baby, to increase blood flow, and to create a healthy environment for your child to grow. Each pound gained is a sign of your body's ability to support life.

- Celebrate Your Bump: Many women feel self-conscious about their growing bellies, but it's important to see your bump as a symbol of strength and life. Embrace your baby bump and find joy in watching it grow. By celebrating your belly, you can feel more connected to the process of pregnancy and develop a deeper appreciation for your body's capabilities.

2. Appreciating Your Body's Strength

Pregnancy is a physically demanding time, and it's easy to focus solely on the outward changes, such as stretch marks or swelling. However, it's equally important to recognize the strength your body is demonstrating. Your body is adapting, expanding, and working hard to support the development of your baby. By appreciating this strength, you can cultivate a sense of pride in your body's resilience.

- Practice Gratitude for Your Body: One way to appreciate your body's strength is by practicing gratitude. Take a few moments each day to reflect on what your body is doing for you and your baby. This could be something as simple as feeling thankful for your legs that carry you, your growing belly that nurtures your baby, or your skin that stretches to accommodate new life.

- Re-frame Physical Changes as Power: Instead of viewing physical changes as losses (such as the loss of a toned stomach or smooth skin), re-frame these changes as a demonstration of your body's power. Stretch marks, swelling, and changes in shape are signs that your body is doing exactly what it needs to do to support pregnancy. By focusing on the powerful aspects of these changes, you can shift your mindset from one of insecurity to one of empowerment.

3. Building a Supportive Community

The journey of pregnancy can be emotionally complex, but you don't have to navigate it alone. Building a supportive community of friends, family, or other expectant mothers can help you feel more positive about your changing body. By sharing your experiences with others who are going through the same process, you'll feel less isolated and more empowered to embrace the changes.

- Join Online or In-Person Groups: Many women find comfort in joining pregnancy support groups, either online or in person. These groups provide a safe space to discuss your thoughts and feelings about body changes and to share tips for staying positive during pregnancy. Connecting with other pregnant women who are experiencing the same challenges can help normalize your feelings and provide emotional support.

- Seek Encouragement from Loved Ones: Don't hesitate to lean on your partner, family members, or close friends for emotional support. They can offer encouragement and remind you of how amazing your body is for carrying life. Sometimes hearing positive affirmations from loved ones can help reinforce your own feelings of self-worth.

How Maternity Fashion Can Boost Your Self-Confidence

What you wear during pregnancy can have a significant impact on how you feel about your body. Wearing clothes that fit well, flatter your growing shape, and reflect your personal style can help boost your confidence and make you feel more comfortable in your changing body. Maternity fashion is designed to provide both comfort and style, ensuring that you feel good about how you look at every stage of pregnancy.

1. Choosing Clothes That Highlight Your Bump

One of the easiest ways to boost your confidence during pregnancy is by embracing clothes that highlight your bump. Rather than hiding your belly under oversize, shapeless clothing, choose maternity pieces that flatter your figure and make you feel proud of your body.

- Fitted Maternity Dresses: Fitted maternity dresses are a great way to celebrate your growing bump. Look for dresses with side ruching or empire waistlines that provide a comfortable fit while accentuating your belly. These styles highlight your bump in a flattering way and can help you feel more connected to the beauty of your pregnant body.

- Belly Bands and Belts: Belly bands and maternity belts can be a great addition to your wardrobe, as they allow you to continue wearing your pre-pregnancy jeans or pants while accommodating your growing belly. Additionally, belts worn just below the bust can help define your silhouette, providing a flattering and stylish look that highlights your pregnancy curves.

2. Prioritizing Comfort Without Sacrificing Style

Many women associate maternity clothes with boring or unflattering designs, but this doesn't have to be the case. Today's maternity fashion offers a wide range of stylish, trendy, and comfortable options that allow you to maintain your personal style throughout pregnancy. Prioritizing comfort doesn't mean sacrificing style—you can have both.

- Stretchy, Breathable Fabrics: When shopping for maternity clothes, look for pieces made from stretchy, breathable fabrics like cotton, jersey, and spandex. These materials provide flexibility and comfort while also maintaining a sleek, stylish appearance. Whether you're wearing maternity leggings, dresses, or tops, choosing fabrics that allow you to move comfortably will help you feel good in your clothes.

- Layering for Versatility: Layering is a great way to stay stylish while ensuring that you're comfortable. Pair a fitted maternity dress with a lightweight cardigan or jacket, or wear a stretchy tank top under an open-front sweater. Layering not only adds dimension to your outfit but also allows you to adjust for changes in temperature, which can be especially helpful during pregnancy when you may feel warmer than usual.

3. Dressing for Your Personality

Just because your body is changing doesn't mean you have to change your sense of style. In fact, dressing in a way that reflects your personality can boost your confidence and help you feel more like yourself during pregnancy. Whether you prefer bold prints, minimalist designs, or something in between, finding maternity clothes that align with your personal style will make you feel more comfortable in your own skin.

- Bold Prints and Colors: If you love bold prints and colors, don't shy away from them during pregnancy. Many maternity brands offer a variety of colorful and patterned pieces that allow you to express your unique sense of style. Wearing bright, fun colors can lift your mood and help you feel more confident about your appearance.

- Accessorizing for Confidence: Accessories like scarves, jewelry, and belts can make a big difference in how you feel about your maternity outfit. Adding a statement necklace or a pair of earrings can transform a simple maternity dress into a polished, stylish look. Don't be afraid to accessorize and experiment with different styles during pregnancy—it's a great way to maintain your sense of individuality.

Dealing with Body Image Issues in Pregnancy

While pregnancy can be a beautiful and empowering experience, it's not uncommon for women to struggle with body image issues during this time. The rapid physical changes, weight gain, and societal pressures to "bounce back" after pregnancy can contribute to feelings of insecurity or frustration. Learning to address and manage these body image concerns is crucial for maintaining a positive and healthy mindset during pregnancy.

1. Acknowledge and Accept Your Feelings

The first step in dealing with body image issues during pregnancy is acknowledging your feelings and accepting that it's okay to have mixed emotions. While many women feel excited and empowered by their pregnancy, it's also normal to feel self-conscious or uncomfortable with the changes happening to your body.

- Validate Your Experience: It's important to remember that your feelings about your body are valid. Pregnancy is a significant change, and it's normal to have moments of discomfort or insecurity. Allow yourself to feel these emotions without judgment and recognize that they don't diminish the beauty of your pregnancy.

- Talk About It: If you're struggling with body image issues, don't hesitate to talk about it with someone you trust. Sharing your thoughts and concerns with a supportive friend, partner, or counselor can help you process your feelings and gain perspective. Often, just knowing that you're not alone in your experience can provide relief.

2. Practice Self-Compassion

One of the most effective ways to deal with body image issues during pregnancy is to practice self-compassion. Your body is going through incredible changes, and it's important to treat yourself with kindness and understanding during this time.

- Speak Kindly to Yourself: Replace negative self-talk with compassionate, positive affirmations. For example, instead of focusing on what you perceive as flaws, remind yourself of how strong and capable your body is for growing new life. Affirmations like "My body is beautiful and powerful" or "I am proud of what my body is doing" can help shift your mindset toward one of self-love and gratitude.

- Set Realistic Expectations: It's easy to get caught up in comparing yourself to others, especially when images of pregnant celebrities or influences flood social media. However, it's important to remember that everyone's pregnancy journey is different. Set realistic expectations for yourself and focus on your unique experience rather than comparing your body to someone else's.

3. Create Healthy Boundaries Around Media Consumption

The media often portrays unrealistic standards of beauty and pregnancy, which can exacerbate body image issues. If you find that certain magazines, social media accounts, or advertisements are making you feel insecure, it may be time to set boundaries around your media consumption.

- Limit Exposure to Harmful Content: Take a break from following accounts or media sources that promote unattainable beauty standards or make you feel less confident about your body. Instead, surround yourself with content that celebrates body positivist, diversity, and real experiences of pregnancy. There are many social media accounts and blogs dedicated to authentic motherhood and body positivist that can provide encouragement and a more balanced perspective.

- Curate Positive Influences: Follow influences, bloggers, or communities that embrace body positivist and self-love during pregnancy. Seeing real women share their honest pregnancy experiences can be incredibly empowering and help you feel more connected to your body. Look for content that uplifts, educates, and celebrates the diversity of pregnancy bodies.

4. Focus on Health Over Appearance

During pregnancy, it's essential to prioritize your health and well-being over societal standards of appearance. Instead of focusing on how your body looks, shift your attention to how you feel and how well you are taking care of yourself and your baby.

- Nourish Your Body: Eating nutritious foods, staying hydrated, and exercising gently are all ways to support your health and feel good during pregnancy. Rather than obsessing over weight or size, focus on giving your body what it needs to thrive during this special time.

- Engage in Gentle Exercise: Physical activity, such as walking, prenatal yoga, or swimming, can boost your mood, reduce stress, and help you feel more connected to your body. Exercise during pregnancy isn't about achieving a certain look—it's about maintaining your physical and mental well-being.

5. Seek Professional Support if Needed

If you find that body image issues are seriously affecting your mental health or your ability to enjoy your pregnancy, it's important to seek professional support. A therapist, counselor, or support group can provide valuable tools and strategies to help you manage body image concerns during pregnancy.

- Cognitive Behavioral Therapy (CBT): CBT is a common therapeutic approach used to treat body image issues. It helps individuals identify and challenge negative thought patterns, replacing them with healthier, more balanced perspectives. If your body image concerns are causing significant distress, a therapist trained in CBT can help you work through these feelings in a constructive way.

- Pregnancy Support Groups: Sometimes, simply talking to other pregnant women who are going through similar experiences can be incredibly helpful. Support groups provide a space to share your feelings, receive encouragement, and connect with others who understand what you're going through.

Pregnancy is an extraordinary journey, both physically and emotionally, and it's natural to experience a wide range of feelings about your changing body. However, by practicing body positivist and focusing on the incredible strength and power of your body, you can build confidence and embrace the beauty of this trans-formative time.

From celebrating your growing belly to dressing in ways that make you feel good, there are many tools you can use to boost your self-confidence during pregnancy. Remember that every woman's pregnancy experience is unique, and there's no right or wrong way to feel about your body as it changes. What's most important is that you approach yourself with kindness, patience, and self-compassion.

Dealing with body image issues is a common challenge, but it's one that can be managed by setting realistic expectations, practicing self-care, and seeking support when needed. By focusing on health, surrounding yourself with positive influences, and creating a supportive environment, you can foster a positive relationship with your body throughout pregnancy and beyond.

Ultimately, your body is performing a remarkable task—creating life. Embracing the changes, challenges, and beauty of pregnancy can lead to a more empowered and joyful experience.

Self-Care Tips for Stylish Moms-to-Be

Pregnancy is a time of immense joy and anticipation, but it also brings with it physical and emotional challenges. As your body undergoes rapid changes to support the growing life inside you, it's essential to prioritize self-care to ensure both comfort and confidence. Maintaining a sense of style and wellness during pregnancy can make you feel more empowered and connected to your evolving body.

In this chapter, we'll explore how to create a self-care routine that supports both comfort and beauty during pregnancy. From essential wellness items like maternity pillows and compression socks to pregnancy-safe skincare products and beauty tips for your hair, skin, and nails, you'll discover a holistic approach to taking care of yourself as a stylish mom-to-be.

Comfort and Wellness Essentials: From Maternity Pillows to Compression Socks

As your body changes during pregnancy, it's important to focus on comfort and wellness to alleviate discomforts such as back pain, swelling, and poor sleep. There are several must-have items that can help support your physical well-being and enhance your quality of life during pregnancy.

1. Maternity Pillows for Better Sleep

Getting a good night's sleep can be difficult during pregnancy, especially as your belly grows and your usual sleeping positions become uncomfortable. A maternity pillow is one of the best investments you can make for your comfort during pregnancy. These specially designed pillows provide support for your back, belly, and hips, helping to alleviate pressure and improve sleep quality.

- Full-Body Maternity Pillows: Full-body maternity pillows are one of the most popular options because they cradle your entire body, providing support from head to toe. These pillows are typically U-shaped or C-shaped and help align your spine, relieve pressure on your hips, and support your growing belly. Full-body pillows are ideal for side sleepers, which is the recommended sleeping position during pregnancy.

- Wedge Pillows: If you prefer a smaller, more versatile pillow, a wedge pillow is a great choice. These compact pillows are designed to fit under your belly or back, providing targeted support where you need it most. Wedge pillows can also be used to elevate your legs, which helps reduce swelling and improves circulation.

- Adjustable Pillows: For moms-to-be who need customized support, adjustable maternity pillows are a flexible option. These pillows often come with removable sections or inserts that allow you to adjust the shape and firmness of the pillow to suit your needs. This makes them perfect for women who want personalized comfort throughout the different stages of pregnancy.

2. Compression Socks for Swelling and Circulation

Swelling in the feet and ankles, known as edema, is a common issue during pregnancy, particularly in the later stages. This happens because your body retains more fluid during pregnancy, and the extra weight puts pressure on your veins, making it harder for blood to circulate. Compression socks are a simple but effective way to alleviate swelling and improve circulation.

- Graduated Compression Socks: These socks are designed with varying levels of pressure, with the strongest compression at the ankle and gradually decreasing up the leg. This helps encourage blood flow back up to the heart and prevents fluid from pooling in the lower extremities. Wearing graduated compression socks during the day can reduce swelling and discomfort, especially if you spend long periods standing or sitting.

- Maternity-Specific Compression Leggings: For moms-to-be who prefer more comprehensive coverage, maternity compression leggings are a great alternative. These leggings provide gentle compression to the legs while also supporting the belly. Many maternity leggings are designed with moisture-wicking fabric to keep you cool and comfortable throughout the day.

- When to Wear Compression Socks: Compression socks are most beneficial when worn during activities that involve prolonged standing or sitting, such as at work, during travel, or even while exercising. It's important to put them on early in the day before swelling starts, as they are most effective at preventing fluid retention when used proactively.

3. Supportive Maternity Bras

As your breasts grow and become more sensitive during pregnancy, it's important to wear bras that offer both support and comfort. Maternity bras are designed to accommodate changes in breast size while providing gentle support for your back and shoulders.

- Wireless Bras: Many moms-to-be find wireless bras to be the most comfortable option during pregnancy. These bras provide support without the discomfort of underwire, which can dig into the skin or cause irritation as your breasts grow. Look for wireless bras with wide straps and a supportive band to ensure adequate lift and comfort.

- Nursing Bras: If you plan to breastfeed, consider investing in nursing bras that can be worn during pregnancy and postpartum. These bras have convenient clips or panels that allow for easy access when breastfeeding, and they often have extra room to accommodate fluctuations in breast size.

- Sleep Bras: Sleep bras are lightweight, stretchy bras designed to provide gentle support while you sleep. They are especially helpful in the later stages of pregnancy when breast tenderness and sensitivity can make it uncomfortable to sleep without support.

Skin Care Tips for Pregnant Women: Choosing Safe Products

Pregnancy can bring about a variety of skin changes, from increased sensitivity to the appearance of stretch marks or acne. Because your skin is more delicate during this time, it's essential to choose products that are both effective and safe for you and your baby. Not all skincare products are suitable for pregnant women, so understanding which ingredients to avoid and which to embrace is key to maintaining healthy, glowing skin.

1. Ingredients to Avoid During Pregnancy

Some common skincare ingredients can be harmful to pregnant women, as they may be absorbed into the bloodstream and potentially affect the baby. Here are some key ingredients to avoid during pregnancy:

- Retinoids (Vitamin A Derivatives): Retinoids, commonly found in anti-aging products, have been linked to birth defects when used in high doses. Avoid products containing retinoids, retinol, or retinoic acid during pregnancy. Opt for safer alternatives, such as bakuchiol, which provides similar anti-aging benefits without the risks.

- Salicylic Acid: High concentrations of salicylic acid, often found in acne treatments, should be avoided during pregnancy. While small amounts in facial cleansers are generally considered safe, it's best to consult your doctor before using products containing salicylic acid. Instead, try gentle exfoliants like lactic acid or glycolic acid for acne-prone skin.

- Hydroquinone: This skin-lightening agent is used to treat hyperpigmentation and melasma (dark spots), but it should be avoided during pregnancy due to the high rate of absorption. For treating pregnancy-related melasma, consider safer options like azelaic acid or vitamin C.

2. Safe and Effective Ingredients for Pregnancy

While some ingredients are off-limits during pregnancy, there are plenty of safe and effective alternatives that can help you maintain healthy skin without compromising the safety of your baby.

- Hyaluronic Acid: Hyaluronic acid is a safe and hydrating ingredient that helps plump and moisturize the skin. It's especially beneficial during pregnancy when hormonal changes can cause dryness. Hyaluronic acid is gentle enough to be used daily and can help maintain the skin's moisture barrier.

- Vitamin C: Vitamin C is a powerful antioxidant that brightens the skin and helps reduce pigmentation. It's safe to use during pregnancy and can be effective in treating pregnancy-related hyperpigmentation or melasma. Incorporate a vitamin C serum into your skincare routine to maintain a radiant complexion.

- Shea Butter and Cocoa Butter: These rich, natural moisturizers are commonly used to prevent and treat stretch marks during pregnancy. Both shea butter and cocoa butter are safe to use and provide deep hydration, which helps keep the skin elastic as it stretches. Regularly applying these butters to areas prone to stretch marks, such as the belly, thighs, and breasts, can help reduce their appearance.

- Zinc Oxide Sunscreen: Protecting your skin from the sun is crucial during pregnancy, as your skin can become more sensitive to UV rays. Choose a mineral sunscreen with zinc oxide or titanium dioxide, as these ingredients sit on top of the skin and reflect UV rays without being absorbed into the bloodstream.

Practicing Self-Care: Hair, Skin, and Nails While Pregnant

Pregnancy hormones can also have a significant impact on the health and appearance of your hair, skin, and nails. While some women experience the "pregnancy glow" and thicker hair, others may deal with skin issues or brittle nails. Maintaining a self-care routine that nurtures these areas can help you feel confident and beautiful throughout your pregnancy.

1. Hair Care During Pregnancy

Hormonal changes during pregnancy can affect your hair in various ways. Many women experience thicker, fuller hair due to increased estrogen levels, which prolong the growth phase of the hair cycle. However, some women may experience hair dryness or changes in texture. Here's how to care for your hair during pregnancy:

- Use Gentle, Hydrating Shampoos: To keep your hair healthy and hydrated, choose shampoos and conditioners that are free of harsh chemicals like sulfates and parabens. Opt for moisturizing formulas that nourish your scalp and hair without stripping away natural oils.

- Scalp Massage for Relaxation and Growth: A gentle scalp massage can stimulate blood flow to the hair follicles, promoting hair growth and providing relaxation. Use your fingertips to massage your scalp in circular motions while shampooing or apply a nourishing hair oil before bed to give your hair extra hydration.

- Avoid Harsh Chemical Treatments: During pregnancy, it's best to avoid chemical treatments like perms, relaxers, and bleach, as the scalp can be more sensitive, and there is limited research on the safety of these treatments during pregnancy. If you're concerned about your hair color, ask your stylist about safer options like highlights or plant-based dyes.

2. Nail Care for Strong and Healthy Nails

Pregnancy hormones can also affect your nails, making them grow faster but potentially more brittle or prone to splitting. To keep your nails strong and healthy during pregnancy, it's essential to focus on nourishing them from the inside out, as well as practicing good nail care habits.

- Moisturize Your Cuticles: Just like your skin, your nails and cuticles can become dry during pregnancy. Regularly applying a cuticle oil or hand cream can keep your nails moisturized and prevent cracking or peeling. This simple step helps maintain the health and appearance of your nails, especially if they are prone to dryness.

- Eat a Balanced Diet: Your nails reflect your overall health, and a balanced diet rich in vitamins and minerals can promote strong, healthy nail growth. Focus on eating foods high in biotin, calcium, and omega-3 fatty acids, such as leafy greens, nuts, seeds, eggs, and fish. These nutrients contribute to nail strength and reduce brittleness.

- Avoid Harsh Nail Products: Steer clear of nail products containing harsh chemicals like formaldehyde, toluene, and dibutyl phthalate (DBP), which are found in some nail polishes and removers. Instead, opt for non-toxic or pregnancy-safe nail products. Many brands now offer "5-free" or "7-free" formulas, which eliminate harmful ingredients from their polishes.

- Trim and File Regularly: Keeping your nails trimmed and filed can prevent breakage and keep them looking neat. If you experience brittle or splitting nails during pregnancy, try using a glass or crystal nail file, which is gentler on the nails compared to traditional emery boards.

3. Skincare for That Pregnancy Glow

While the famous "pregnancy glow" is often attributed to increased blood circulation and hormonal changes, not every woman experiences flawless skin during pregnancy. Hormonal fluctuations can lead to breakouts, dryness, and increased sensitivity. A good skincare routine can help address these concerns and keep your skin looking its best.

- Hydration is Key: Staying hydrated is one of the simplest and most effective ways to maintain healthy skin during pregnancy. Drinking plenty of water helps your skin stay supple and reduces the likelihood of dryness. In addition to drinking water, using a hydrating serum or moisturizer can lock in moisture and keep your skin looking plump.

- Gentle Exfoliation: Hormonal changes can lead to an increase in dead skin cells, making your skin look dull or congested. Gentle exfoliation can help remove these dead cells and reveal brighter, smoother skin. Choose a mild exfoliant, like a lactic acid or enzyme-based product, to slough away dead skin without irritating your more sensitive pregnancy skin.

- Treating Acne During Pregnancy: Acne can sometimes worsen during pregnancy due to hormonal surges. If you're experiencing breakouts, it's important to use products that are safe for pregnancy. Benzoyl peroxide and salicylic acid should be avoided in high concentrations, but products containing sulfur or azelaic acid are safer alternatives for treating acne.

4. Self-Care for Emotional Well-Being

In addition to physical self-care, emotional well-being is a crucial part of feeling confident and radiant during pregnancy. Pregnancy can bring about a range of emotions, from excitement to anxiety, and it's essential to create time for self-care practices that support your mental health.

- Meditation and Mindfulness: Pregnancy is a time of heightened emotions and stress, so incorporating mindfulness or meditation into your routine can help you stay grounded. Simple practices like deep breathing, guided meditation, or even journaling can reduce anxiety and promote a sense of calm.

- Prenatal Yoga: Prenatal yoga is an excellent way to combine physical and emotional self-care. Not only does it help keep your body flexible and strong, but it also provides a space to connect with your baby and focus on relaxation. Many prenatal yoga classes incorporate breathing exercises and meditation, which can help alleviate stress and improve your overall sense of well-being.

- Pampering Sessions: Don't underestimate the power of pampering yourself. Whether it's a warm bath with Epsom salts, a gentle facial massage, or a DIY manicure, taking time to pamper yourself can boost your mood and help you feel more relaxed. Create a self-care routine that allows you to unwind and indulge in small luxuries that make you feel good.

5. Maintaining Personal Style While Practicing Self-Care

Looking stylish and feeling comfortable can go hand in hand during pregnancy. Many women feel a boost of confidence when they wear clothes that reflect their personal style, and this extends to how you care for your hair, skin, and nails. Finding balance between self-care and style is key to feeling like your best self during pregnancy.

- Simplify Your Beauty Routine: Pregnancy is the perfect time to streamline your beauty routine. Focus on products and routines that work for your changing body without overwhelming your schedule. For example, a multitasking product like a tinted moisturizer with SPF can simplify your makeup routine while providing sun protection and hydration.

- Embrace a Low-Maintenance Hair Routine: Many women find that pregnancy gives their hair extra volume and shine, but if you're dealing with dryness or texture changes, opt for a low-maintenance routine that keeps your hair healthy. Regular trims, deep conditioning treatments, and air-drying your hair can all help reduce stress on your hair and scalp.

- Choose Comfort and Confidence in Fashion: When dressing during pregnancy, it's important to choose outfits that make you feel both comfortable and confident. Invest in a few high-quality, versatile maternity pieces that suit your personal style, such as well-fitting leggings, a chic maternity dress, and comfortable flats. Pair these with your favorite accessories to maintain your signature look while accommodating your growing bump.

Self-care during pregnancy goes beyond comfort—it's about nurturing your body, mind, and spirit as you navigate this exciting and trans-formative time. By incorporating wellness essentials like maternity pillows and compression socks, choosing pregnancy-safe skincare products, and maintaining a self-care routine for your hair, skin, and nails, you can feel confident and beautiful throughout your pregnancy journey.

Taking care of yourself not only enhances your sense of style but also supports your emotional well-being, helping you stay grounded and connected to your body as it changes. Whether it's through investing in high-quality beauty products, practicing mindfulness, or simply indulging in a relaxing bath, self-care is an essential part of feeling empowered and radiant as a mom-to-be.

Ultimately, self-care during pregnancy is about celebrating your body's incredible abilities, prioritizing your comfort and well-being, and maintaining your unique sense of style. By focusing on both wellness and beauty, you can create a pregnancy experience that is as stylish as it is fulfilling, allowing you to embrace this special time with confidence and joy.

Celebrity Maternity Style: Inspiration from Famous Moms

Celebrities have long been a source of inspiration for fashion, and maternity style is no exception. From red-carpet gowns to street style, famous moms-to-be have a way of making pregnancy look glamorous, confident, and effortlessly chic. Their fashion choices have a significant influence on maternity trends, and many expectant mothers look to these stars for ideas on how to dress their growing bumps.

In this chapter, we will explore how celebrities stay stylish during pregnancy, the maternity fashion trends influenced by famous moms, and how you can adapt these celebrity-inspired looks to fit your own budget and comfort. Whether you're looking to channel the elegance of a red-carpet ensemble or the casual coolness of everyday celebrity wear, there are plenty of ways to incorporate these styles into your maternity wardrobe without breaking the bank.

How Celebrities Stay Stylish During Pregnancy

Many celebrities manage to maintain their personal style throughout pregnancy, whether it's by adapting their pre-pregnancy wardrobe or experimenting with new, maternity-specific pieces. Celebrity moms have access to the world's top designers and stylists, but their fashion choices often follow universal principles that can be adopted by anyone.

1. Embracing Body Confidence and Celebrating the Bump

One of the most noticeable aspects of celebrity maternity fashion is the confidence with which these women embrace their changing bodies. Rather than hiding their bumps under oversize clothing, many famous moms-to-be proudly show off their growing bellies in form-fitting outfits that accentuate their pregnancy curves.

- Fitted Silhouettes: Celebrities like Blake Lively, Kim Kardashian, and Chrissy Teigen have all been known to wear fitted dresses and jumpsuits that hug their bumps. These silhouettes celebrate the body's changing shape and project confidence. For women who feel comfortable showing off their bump, fitted maternity dresses or body-hugging outfits can help you feel more connected to the beauty of your pregnant body.

- Sheer and Transparent Fabrics: Another trend in celebrity maternity fashion is the use of sheer fabrics that subtly reveal the bump. Celebrities like Beyoncé and Rihanna have embraced transparent or semi-sheer gowns on the red carpet, giving a glamorous peek at their baby bump while maintaining a sense of elegance. While sheer fabrics may not be for everyone, they offer a way to celebrate the bump while still feeling stylish and fashion-forward.

- Crop Tops and Two-Piece Sets: Celebrities like Rihanna have challenged traditional maternity fashion by wearing bold crop tops or two-piece sets that highlight the bump. This edgy look showcases the belly with pride and brings a modern twist to maternity wear. If you're feeling adventurous, a two-piece set or crop top can be paired with a high-waited skirt or maternity pants for a look that is both fun and fashion-forward.

2. Mixing Maternity and Non-Maternity Pieces

One of the secrets to celebrity maternity style is that many famous moms-to-be don't rely solely on maternity-specific clothing. Instead, they often mix maternity pieces with non-maternity items from their pre-pregnancy wardrobe, creating a look that stays true to their personal style.

- Over-sized Blazers and Coats: Celebrities like Meghan Markle and Gigi Hadid have often been seen wearing oversize blazers, trench coats, and outerwear during pregnancy. These pieces are perfect for layering over fitted maternity dresses or leggings, adding a polished look while accommodating a growing belly. Blazers and coats with a looser fit offer flexibility and can be worn throughout pregnancy and beyond.

- Stretchy Fabrics and Flowy Dresses: Flowy dresses and stretchy fabrics are a staple in many celebrity maternity wardrobes. These pieces can easily accommodate a growing bump without sacrificing style. Look for non-maternity items like wrap dresses, maxi dresses, or empire-waist dresses that provide room for your belly and can transition into postpartum wear.

- Accessories for Versatility: Accessories play a key role in transforming an outfit, and celebrities often rely on bold accessories to elevate their maternity style. From statement belts to bold jewelry, adding a few eye-catching accessories can help tie together a maternity look while staying on-trend. Belts worn just above the bump can help define your waistline, while scarves, hats, and oversize sunglasses add personality to a simple maternity outfit.

3. Red-Carpet Glamour

While many of us don't attend red-carpet events during pregnancy, there's no denying that celebrity moms-to-be often steal the show with their glamorous, high-fashion maternity looks. Red-carpet maternity fashion is all about making a statement, and many celebrities use this opportunity to showcase custom-made gowns, designer dresses, and luxurious fabrics.

- Bold Colors and Statement Gowns: Celebrities like Cardi B, Blake Lively, and Serena Williams have embraced bold, statement-making gowns during their pregnancies. From bright, eye-catching colors to voluminous tulle skirts, these red-carpet looks are designed to turn heads. If you have a special event during your pregnancy, you can take inspiration from these bold looks by opting for a colorful gown or a maternity dress with dramatic details like ruffles, sequins, or embellishments.

- Elegant Draping and Silhouettes: Red-carpet looks often feature elegant draping, flowing fabrics, and figure-flattering silhouettes that highlight the baby bump. Celebrities like Jessica Alba and Natalie Port man have opted for gowns with empire waists or flowing skirts, creating a romantic and ethereal look. For more formal occasions, consider choosing a gown with soft, draped fabric that provides comfort while still offering a glamorous appearance.

- Custom Couture and Tailoring: Many celebrity moms have their maternity looks custom-made by top designers, ensuring a perfect fit for their growing bodies. While custom couture may be out of reach for most of us, tailoring can make a big difference in how your maternity clothes fit. Consider taking your favorite pieces to a tailor to ensure they flatter your shape, especially as your body continues to change throughout pregnancy.

Maternity Fashion Trends Influenced by Celebrities

Celebrities play a significant role in shaping fashion trends, and maternity wear is no exception. Over the years, many celebrity moms have popularized new styles, designs, and fabrics that have become staples in maternity fashion. These trends are often embraced by expectant mothers around the world, influencing the way women dress during pregnancy.

1. The Rise of Athleisure and Comfortable Fashion

One of the biggest trends in recent years, both in mainstream and maternity fashion, is athleisure. Celebrities like Gigi Hadid, Kylie Jenner, and Serena Williams have all embraced comfortable, athletic-inspired clothing during their pregnancies, showing that you don't have to sacrifice style for comfort. The athleisure trend combines functionality with fashion, making it easy for pregnant women to feel both comfortable and stylish.

- Maternity Leggings and Joggers: Maternity leggings and joggers have become a staple in many women's pregnancy wardrobes, thanks to their comfort and versatility. These pieces can be worn for casual outings, lounging at home, or even light exercise. Look for leggings with over-the-belly support or joggers with adjustable waistbands to accommodate your growing bump.

- Matching Sets: Another trend in athleisure is the rise of matching sets. Celebrities like Kim Kardashian have popularized the look of matching crop tops and leggings or sweatshirts and joggers. This trend is easy to adapt to maternity wear, as many brands now offer matching maternity sets that are both comfortable and stylish.

2. Luxe Lounge-wear

With many celebrities posting photos of themselves at home in luxurious, cozy Lounge-wear, it's no surprise that this trend has made its way into maternity fashion. Famous moms like Ashley Graham and Chrissy Teigen have embraced the look of luxurious robes, soft pajama sets, and cozy knitwear during their pregnancies.

- Silk Robes and Satin Pajamas: Silk robes and satin pajamas have become a popular trend for maternity Lounge-wear, offering a glamorous and comfortable option for moms-to-be. These pieces are perfect for lounging around the house, and they can even transition into postpartum wear for nursing or late-night feedings. Choose fabrics that are soft and breathable, such as silk, satin, or cotton blends, for ultimate comfort.

- Cashmere Sweaters and Knitwear: Cozy knitwear has also made its mark in maternity fashion, thanks to celebrities like Blake Lively and Emily Blunt. Cashmere sweaters, oversize cardigans, and soft knit dresses provide warmth and comfort while maintaining a chic look. Invest in a few high-quality knitwear pieces that can be worn throughout your pregnancy and beyond.

3. Gender-Neutral and Minimalist Styles

In recent years, many celebrities have embraced gender-neutral and minimalist fashion, and this trend has also extended into maternity wear. Celebrity moms like Meghan Markle and Jessica Alba have popularized the idea of simple, minimalist maternity outfits that rely on neutral colors, clean lines, and timeless pieces.

- Neutral Color Palettes: Minimalist maternity fashion often involves neutral color palettes, such as black, white, beige, and gray. These colors are versatile and can be easily mixed and matched to create a range of stylish outfits. For women who prefer a more understated look, a neutral maternity wardrobe can provide the perfect balance of style and simplicity.

- Tailored and Structured Pieces: Minimalist maternity fashion often includes tailored and structured pieces, such as blazers, trench coats, and crisp button-down shirts. These items can add a polished, sophisticated touch to your maternity wardrobe while still being comfortable. Look for pieces that offer flexibility and room for your growing bump without sacrificing structure.

Adapting Celebrity Styles to Fit Your Budget and Comfort

While celebrity maternity fashion may seem glamorous and unattainable, there are plenty of ways to incorporate these trends into your own wardrobe without breaking the bank. With a little creativity and resourcefulness, you can adapt celebrity styles to fit both your budget and your comfort needs. Whether you're inspired by the chic red-carpet looks of famous moms or the laid-back, everyday styles they wear, here are practical tips for bringing those celebrity maternity looks into your wardrobe without spending a fortune.

1. Shop for Budget-Friendly Maternity Pieces

While celebrities often wear designer pieces, many of the maternity trends they popularize can be found at affordable retailers. Look for budget-friendly versions of celebrity-inspired maternity clothing at stores like H&M, Old Navy, ASOS, and Target. These retailers offer stylish, comfortable maternity clothes that follow the latest trends without the high price tag.

- Affordable Dresses and Gowns: If you're inspired by the glamorous red-carpet looks worn by celebrities, you can find affordable maternity dresses that mimic those styles. For special occasions, look for dresses with flowing fabrics, empire waists, or elegant draping that are available at more accessible prices. Many retailers offer affordable yet stylish formal maternity dresses that are perfect for events like baby showers, weddings, or maternity photo-shoots.

- Maternity Athleisure: For those who love the athleisure trend embraced by celebrities, you don't need to spend a lot to get the look. Budget-friendly brands like Gap, Amazon, and Target offer maternity leggings, joggers, and matching sets that combine comfort with style. Look for pieces made from soft, stretchy fabrics that provide support for your growing bump.

2. Mix Maternity and Non-Maternity Clothing

Just like many celebrities, you don't have to rely solely on maternity-specific clothing to stay stylish during pregnancy. Many non-maternity pieces, particularly those made from stretchy or flowy fabrics, can be worn throughout your pregnancy and even postpartum. By mixing maternity and non-maternity pieces, you can extend your wardrobe and make your outfits more versatile.

- Invest in Key Maternity Staples: Invest in a few high-quality maternity staples, such as maternity leggings, jeans, and fitted dresses, and then pair them with non-maternity items from your existing wardrobe. For example, you can wear an oversize blazer or a long cardigan from your pre-pregnancy closet over a fitted maternity dress to create a chic, layered look.

- Accessorize to Elevate Your Look: Accessories are an easy way to add a touch of celebrity flair to your maternity outfits. Just like famous moms often use belts, scarves, and jewelry to elevate their looks, you can do the same. Belts worn above your bump can help define your waist, while statement necklaces, earrings, or sunglasses can add personality to a simple maternity outfit.

3. Tailor Your Maternity Clothes

Tailoring is a cost-effective way to ensure that your maternity clothes fit perfectly, just like the custom couture pieces worn by celebrities. By taking your clothes to a tailor, you can make minor adjustments that improve the fit and make your outfits more flattering. This is particularly helpful for special occasions when you want to look your best.

- Customize Off-the-Rack Pieces: You don't need to buy expensive designer maternity clothes to get a tailored look. Off-the-rack maternity clothes from affordable retailers can be tailored to fit your body better. For example, you can have a dress taken in at the sides, or a pair of pants adjusted for a more comfortable fit. Tailoring can make even budget-friendly clothes look and feel high-end.

- Re-purpose Non-Maternity Clothes: If you're wearing non-maternity clothes that you want to continue using during pregnancy, a tailor can help adjust them to accommodate your growing bump. For example, a tailor can add extra fabric to the sides of a dress or adjust the waistband of a skirt or pants for a more comfortable fit.

4. Embrace Thrift Shopping and Secondhand Options

If you're looking to replicate celebrity maternity styles on a tight budget, thrift shopping and secondhand stores are excellent options. Many women sell or donate their maternity clothes after giving birth, so you can find gently used, high-quality pieces at a fraction of the cost of buying new.

- Consignment Stores: Many consignment stores specialize in maternity and baby clothing, offering a wide range of stylish, gently used maternity wear. You can often find designer pieces at a steep discount, making it possible to achieve a celebrity-inspired look without spending a lot.

- Online Secondhand Platforms: Platforms like Posh mark, ThredUP, and Facebook Marketplace allow you to browse and buy secondhand maternity clothes online. These platforms often feature popular maternity brands and designer pieces, allowing you to score celebrity-inspired outfits at more affordable prices.

5. DIY Fashion Hacks for Maternity Style

If you're feeling creative, you can make your own alterations or up-cycle pieces from your wardrobe to create celebrity-inspired maternity looks. DIY fashion hacks allow you to personalize your clothes and save money while staying stylish during pregnancy.

- Add Side Panels to Dresses or Tops: One simple DIY hack is adding stretchy side panels to non-maternity dresses or tops to make them bump-friendly. This allows you to continue wearing your favorite pre-pregnancy clothes while accommodating your growing belly.

- Turn Regular Pants into Maternity Pants: If you want to keep wearing your pre-pregnancy jeans or pants, you can add a stretchy belly panel or use a belly band to make them more comfortable. Belly bands are an inexpensive and easy way to extend the life of your pre-pregnancy pants without buying new maternity clothes.

While celebrities may have access to high-end designers and personal stylists, their approach to maternity fashion offers plenty of inspiration for moms-to-be at any budget level. From body-hugging dresses and athleisure trends to tailored pieces and luxe Lounge-wear, the key to celebrity maternity style is confidence, comfort, and creativity.

By mixing maternity and non-maternity pieces, investing in key staples, and using accessories to elevate your outfits, you can create a maternity wardrobe that's both stylish and practical. Whether you're inspired by the red-carpet glamour of famous moms or the everyday chic of athleisure, there are countless ways to adapt celebrity maternity trends to fit your personal style, budget, and comfort needs.

Ultimately, the most important aspect of maternity fashion is feeling good in your own skin. As your body changes and grows, embrace the process with confidence and pride, just like your favorite celebrity moms. By taking inspiration from their bold fashion choices and adapting them to your lifestyle, you can stay stylish and empowered throughout your pregnancy journey.

Chapter 18: Maternity Fashion Trends: What's Hot Right Now?

Maternity fashion has come a long way in recent years, with more options than ever for moms-to-be who want to stay on-trend while ensuring comfort. As we move into 2024, maternity fashion trends are evolving to embrace both functionality and style, blending the latest runway trends with the practical needs of pregnancy. Whether you're looking for bold, fashion-forward pieces or timeless staples that will serve you well beyond pregnancy, understanding the key trends of the moment can help you craft a maternity wardrobe that reflects your unique sense of style.

In this chapter, we'll dive into the hottest maternity fashion trends for 2024, offer advice on how to incorporate these trends into your everyday wardrobe, and explore how to strike a balance between trendy and timeless pieces. With a thoughtful approach, you can look and feel your best throughout your pregnancy while staying true to your personal style.

Current Maternity Fashion Trends for 2024

In 2024, maternity fashion is all about blending comfort with style. Many of the trends seen in mainstream fashion have seamlessly transitioned into the maternity space, giving expectant mothers more options than ever to express their individuality. These trends emphasize the importance of self-care, body positivist, and versatility, allowing pregnant women to feel confident and comfortable no matter the occasion.

1. Sustainable and Eco-Friendly Maternity Fashion

As sustainability continues to be a major focus in the fashion industry, eco-friendly maternity wear is one of the hottest trends for 2024. Many expecting mothers are now prioritizing sustainable, ethical fashion choices that align with their values. Maternity brands are responding by creating eco-conscious collections made from organic cotton, bamboo, and recycled materials. These pieces not only reduce environmental impact but also offer high levels of comfort and breath-ability, which are essential during pregnancy.

- Why It's Trending: Sustainability is no longer a niche movement—it's becoming a mainstream expectation. With more people becoming environ-mentally conscious, expectant mothers are opting for eco-friendly maternity clothes that are ethically produced, long-lasting, and made from natural fibers. Brands like Boob, Seraphine, and Pact are leading the way with collections that emphasize both style and sustainability.

- How to Wear It: Look for maternity essentials made from organic or recycled materials, such as organic cotton leggings, bamboo maternity tops, or sustainable maternity dresses. Many of these pieces are designed to be versatile, making them suitable for both pregnancy and postpartum. Choose neutral colors and timeless cuts that can be mixed and matched, allowing you to build a sustainable, capsule maternity wardrobe.

2. Bold Prints and Patterns

In 2024, bold prints and patterns are making a splash in maternity fashion. From floral and geometric designs to animal prints, expectant mothers are embracing eye-catching patterns that add personality and vibrancy to their maternity wardrobes. Whether you prefer a statement dress in a bold print or subtle accents through accessories, there are plenty of ways to incorporate this trend into your pregnancy style.

- Why It's Trending: Bold prints and patterns are a fun way to express individuality and bring excitement to maternity wear, which is often dominated by neutral colors. With fashion-forward moms wanting to make a statement, prints like leopard, zebra, and oversize florals are becoming a staple in maternity collections. Celebrities and influences have also been spotted in bold maternity prints, further driving the trend.

- How to Wear It: To make bold prints work for your maternity wardrobe, start with one statement piece, such as a printed maxi dress or a patterned maternity blouse. Pair it with more neutral, solid-colored pieces to balance the look. If you're hesitant to wear large prints, try incorporating them through accessories, like a printed scarf or a patterned handbag, for a subtler take on the trend.

3. Athleisure for Pregnancy

Athleisure continues to dominate mainstream fashion, and it's a natural fit for maternity wear in 2024. Expectant mothers are increasingly opting for comfortable, stretchy pieces that can transition from lounging at home to running errands. Maternity athleisure is characterized by soft fabrics, supportive waistbands, and stylish cuts that make it easy to look put-together while staying comfortable. This trend prioritizes flexibility and ease, with pieces like maternity leggings, joggers, and oversize sweatshirts leading the way.

- Why It's Trending: Athleisure's popularity lies in its versatility and comfort, two factors that are especially important for pregnant women. The stretchy, breathable materials used in athleisure make it an ideal choice for women experiencing body changes during pregnancy. Plus, the trend's blend of casual and chic fits easily into modern, on-the-go lifestyles.

- How to Wear It: Incorporate maternity athleisure into your wardrobe by investing in a few high-quality pieces like supportive maternity leggings, oversize hoodies, or maternity-friendly active-wear sets. Look for items made from moisture-wicking fabrics that offer support for your growing belly. You can also elevate your athleisure look by adding accessories like a stylish pair of sneakers or a cross body bag.

4. Luxe Lounge-wear

Luxe Lounge-wear is another major trend in maternity fashion for 2024. Pregnant women are prioritizing comfort without sacrificing style, and luxurious Lounge-wear offers the best of both worlds. Soft fabrics like cashmere, silk, and modal are being used in maternity pajama sets, robes, and lounge dresses, making it easy for moms-to-be to relax at home while still feeling chic. This trend reflects the growing importance of self-care and wellness during pregnancy.

- Why It's Trending: As many people continue to work from home or spend more time indoors, the demand for stylish yet comfortable Lounge-wear has surged. Luxe Lounge-wear allows pregnant women to feel pampered and relaxed, while also offering pieces that can transition from day to night with ease. The rise of "elevated comfort" in fashion has made luxe Lounge-wear a go-to choice for expectant mothers.

- How to Wear It: To incorporate luxe Lounge-wear into your maternity wardrobe, look for pieces made from soft, high-quality fabrics that feel good against your skin. A cashmere maternity cardigan, a silk lounge dress, or a cozy matching pajama set can be both stylish and functional. These pieces are perfect for lounging at home but can also be worn for casual outings when paired with the right accessories.

5. Gender-Neutral Maternity Fashion

As gender-neutral fashion becomes more mainstream, maternity wear is following suit. In 2024, expect to see more gender-neutral maternity pieces that focus on clean lines, simple cuts, and neutral color palettes like black, white, and beige. This trend is all about embracing minimalism and functionality, offering versatile pieces that can be worn by anyone and for any occasion.

- Why It's Trending: Gender-neutral fashion aligns with the growing movement toward inclusivity and sustainability. Expectant mothers who want to move away from traditionally "feminine" maternity wear are gravitating toward minimalistic, versatile pieces that focus on comfort and practicality rather than gendered designs. These pieces are often more timeless and can be easily incorporated into a postpartum wardrobe.

- How to Wear It: Incorporate gender-neutral maternity fashion by choosing pieces with simple, classic cuts and neutral colors. A tailored maternity blazer, a pair of black maternity trousers, or a white button-up shirt can serve as the foundation of a minimalist maternity wardrobe. These pieces can be dressed up or down depending on the occasion and can easily transition into postpartum wear.

6. Dresses with Ruching and Adjustable Features

Ruching has long been a favorite in maternity wear, and it continues to be a key trend in 2024. Dresses with ruching along the sides or adjustable features such as drawstrings and ties are popular because they allow for flexibility as the belly grows. These dresses hug the body in all the right places, flattering the bump while offering room to expand.

- Why It's Trending: Ruching is a practical design element that adds both style and comfort to maternity wear. It helps create a flattering silhouette by providing structure while also accommodating a growing bump. The adjustable features in many maternity dresses make them versatile, allowing moms-to-be to wear them throughout different stages of pregnancy.

- How to Wear It: Ruching works well in both casual and formal maternity dresses. Look for ruched maternity dresses in soft fabrics that allow for plenty of movement and stretch. Dresses with adjustable ties at the waist or sides are also great for creating a customized fit. Pair a ruched dress with simple sandals for a daytime look or dress it up with heels and statement jewelry for an evening event.

Incorporating Trends Into Your Maternity Wardrobe

Incorporating maternity fashion trends into your wardrobe doesn't mean you have to follow every trend. The key is to select trends that resonate with your personal style, comfort needs, and lifestyle. Here are some tips for seamlessly blending maternity fashion trends into your wardrobe:

1. Start with the Basics

Every maternity wardrobe should begin with a few staple pieces that can be mixed and matched with trendier items. Invest in high-quality basics like maternity leggings, jeans, tank tops, and dresses in neutral colors. Once you have a foundation, you can incorporate trendier pieces like bold prints, luxe Lounge-wear, or athleisure to add variety to your outfits.

2. Prioritize Comfort and Functionality

During pregnancy, comfort is paramount. While it can be tempting to follow fashion trends, always prioritize pieces that make you feel comfortable and supported. Trends like athleisure and luxe Lounge-wear are perfect because they offer both style and comfort. Look for fabrics that are breathable and stretchy, ensuring they grow with your bump and keep you feeling at ease throughout the day.

3. Choose Versatile Pieces

When incorporating trends into your maternity wardrobe, it's wise to choose versatile pieces that can be worn in multiple ways and for different occasions. This ensures that you're getting the most out of your clothing, especially since maternity wear is typically worn for a limited time. For example, a bold printed maternity dress can be styled with sneakers for a casual daytime look, or paired with heels and statement jewelry for a more formal event. Versatile pieces like stretchy maternity leggings, wrap dresses, and tunics are perfect for transitioning from day to night or from work to weekend.

4. Mix and Match Trends with Timeless Pieces

One of the best ways to incorporate trends into your maternity wardrobe is to mix trendy items with timeless staples. This allows you to stay fashionable while also building a wardrobe that will last beyond your pregnancy. For example, you might pair a trendy animal print top with classic black maternity trousers, or layer a luxe maternity cardigan over a timeless, ruched dress. By combining trendy items with timeless basics, you can create a balanced, cohesive wardrobe that feels modern but not overly trendy.

5. Don't Be Afraid to Experiment

Pregnancy is the perfect time to experiment with your style and try new trends that you might not have considered before. Whether it's stepping out of your comfort zone with bold prints, trying out gender-neutral clothing, or embracing the athleisure trend, don't be afraid to play around with different looks. Pregnancy is a unique time in your life, and your wardrobe should reflect the excitement and transformation you're experiencing. Have fun with fashion, and remember that maternity trends are designed to make you feel confident, comfortable, and stylish.

Finding Balance Between Trendy and Timeless Maternity Pieces

While it's tempting to follow the latest fashion trends, it's important to strike a balance between trendy and timeless pieces in your maternity wardrobe. Investing in too many trendy items can leave you with a wardrobe full of clothes that may not be practical once your pregnancy is over. On the other hand, filling your wardrobe with only basics might make it feel uninspiring or boring. Here's how to achieve the perfect balance:

1. Build a Capsule Wardrobe

A maternity capsule wardrobe consists of essential, timeless pieces that can be mixed and matched to create multiple outfits. These items should be versatile, comfortable, and suitable for different occasions. Once you have a solid foundation of capsule pieces, you can introduce trendy items that add personality and flair to your wardrobe. Capsule pieces might include:

- Maternity Leggings and Jeans: High-quality leggings and jeans with supportive waistbands are a maternity must-have. Look for neutral colors like black, navy, or dark denim, which can be worn with various tops and accessories.

- Simple Maternity Dresses: A few simple maternity dresses in classic cuts, such as wrap dresses or ruched dresses, can be styled in countless ways. Opt for solid colors like black, gray, or navy, which can be dressed up or down with accessories.

- Basic Tops and Tees: Maternity tops in neutral tones or soft fabrics are essential for layering. Long-sleeve tees, tank tops, and button-up shirts in breathable fabrics will serve as the backbone of your wardrobe.

Once you have these core pieces, you can start incorporating seasonal trends, like bold prints or athleisure, for added variety.

2. Invest in Timeless, Quality Pieces

While it's easy to get caught up in the excitement of trendy maternity fashion, it's important to invest in timeless, quality pieces that you'll wear frequently during your pregnancy. High-quality maternity clothing tends to be more durable, offering better support and comfort as your body changes. For example, a well-made black maternity dress, a tailored blazer, or a pair of comfortable, stretchy jeans are worth the investment because they can be worn multiple times and for different occasions. These items will likely stay in good condition for any future pregnancies as well.

3. Keep Trends Subtle

If you're hesitant about going all-in on trendy maternity pieces, start by incorporating trends in small doses. Accessories, like scarves, shoes, or bags, are an easy way to introduce trends without overhauling your entire wardrobe. You could also choose one or two trendy pieces, like a bold-printed dress or a statement jacket, and pair them with your more classic maternity basics. This approach allows you to enjoy current trends while maintaining a timeless and versatile wardrobe.

4. Consider Post-Pregnancy Wearability

When shopping for trendy maternity pieces, consider whether they'll be useful after pregnancy. Many maternity items can be worn postpartum, especially those with adjustable features or stretchable fabrics. For example, maternity dresses with ruching or wrap-style tops can easily transition into postpartum wear, offering both style and comfort after the baby arrives. Look for pieces that offer flexibility, such as nursing-friendly tops or dresses that can be worn during and after pregnancy.

5. Choose Trends That Reflect Your Personal Style

Not every maternity trend will suit your personal taste, and that's okay. The key to finding balance between trendy and timeless is to choose trends that reflect your style and personality. If bold prints don't feel right for you, stick with more subtle patterns or opt for gender-neutral, minimalist looks. If athleisure is your go-to, embrace that style throughout your pregnancy with leggings and oversize sweatshirts. The goal is to feel comfortable, confident, and true to yourself while staying on-trend.

Maternity fashion in 2024 is all about blending comfort with style. The latest trends—ranging from sustainable fashion to bold prints, athleisure, and luxe Lounge-wear—offer endless opportunities to express your individuality while staying comfortable during pregnancy. By thoughtfully incorporating these trends into your maternity wardrobe, you can stay fashionable without sacrificing functionality.

Finding balance between trendy and timeless pieces is key to building a maternity wardrobe that serves you well throughout pregnancy and beyond. Start by investing in a few high-quality, versatile basics, then layer in trendy pieces to keep your wardrobe fresh and exciting. Most importantly, choose items that reflect your personal style and make you feel confident and empowered.

Whether you're embracing eco-friendly fashion, experimenting with bold patterns, or staying cozy in luxe Lounge-wear, 2024 offers a wide array of maternity fashion options to suit every mom-to-be. By balancing trend-driven styles with timeless staples, you can create a maternity wardrobe that not only keeps you on-trend but also helps you feel your best during this special time in your life.

Conclusion

Pregnancy is a trans-formative experience, both physically and emotionally, and your maternity fashion journey reflects this evolution. As your body changes to accommodate new life, so does your approach to dressing. What once felt stylish may no longer provide the comfort you need, and pieces that were once foreign to your wardrobe may become essentials. Throughout your pregnancy, you've likely had moments of discovery, creativity, and even frustration, but ultimately, your maternity fashion journey is about learning to honor your body and prioritize your well-being.

In this concluding chapter, we'll take a moment to reflect on how your style has evolved during pregnancy, consider how you can continue to dress comfortably and stylishly during the postpartum phase, and share some final thoughts on the role of maternity fashion in enhancing both comfort and confidence.

Reflecting on Your Pregnancy and Style Evolution

Your pregnancy journey has likely been one of the most significant changes your body has ever experienced. Over the course of nine months, your body has transformed in ways that are both visible and invisible. It's natural to feel a mix of emotions as you navigate these changes—sometimes embracing your growing belly with pride, and other times feeling uncertain or disconnected from your pre-pregnancy self. However, your maternity fashion choices have played a key role in helping you feel grounded, comfortable, and stylish throughout the process.

1. Embracing Your Changing Body

At the start of your pregnancy, you may have felt apprehensive about how your body would change and how to dress for it. Perhaps you tried to hold onto your pre-pregnancy wardrobe for as long as possible, relying on loose-fitting tops and stretchy pants. But as your belly grew and your body's needs shifted, you likely found yourself seeking new solutions—whether it was embracing maternity jeans with an over-the-belly band, discovering the comfort of stretchy dresses, or finally finding a maternity bra that provided the support you needed.

Throughout this journey, you've come to embrace your body's changes. You've discovered that maternity fashion isn't just about practicality—it's about celebrating the beauty and power of your body as it nurtures new life. Whether you've leaned into fitted maternity pieces that showcase your bump or opted for flowy, comfortable outfits that provide freedom of movement, your wardrobe has become a reflection of your evolving relationship with your body.

- Celebrating Milestones Through Fashion: Every stage of pregnancy comes with its own set of milestones, and your fashion choices have likely mirrored these moments. Perhaps you bought your first pair of maternity jeans after your belly "popped" or invested in a special dress for your baby shower. These fashion milestones aren't just about the clothes themselves—they're about how you've navigated the physical and emotional changes of pregnancy with grace and confidence.

- Learning to Prioritize Comfort: Early in your pregnancy, you might have prioritized style over comfort, trying to maintain your usual fashion sense. However, as your pregnancy progressed, comfort likely became a top priority. You may have learned to balance both by choosing pieces that make you feel good while also providing the support and flexibility your body needs. This shift in perspective is a natural part of the pregnancy journey, as you learn to honor your body's needs while maintaining a sense of self-expression.

2. Adapting Your Personal Style

Pregnancy often requires you to adapt your personal style in ways you hadn't anticipated. You may have found yourself exploring new trends, trying out silhouettes you wouldn't have considered before, or even experimenting with accessories to elevate a simple maternity outfit. This period of adaptation can be a creative time, allowing you to expand your wardrobe in ways that reflect your evolving identity as a mom-to-be.

- Exploring New Trends: Many pregnant women discover a newfound appreciation for trends like athleisure, gender-neutral clothing, or even bold prints they may not have worn before. Pregnancy is a time when fashion takes on a new form—one that prioritizes both function and style. Whether you embraced maternity leggings, flowy maxi dresses, or luxe Lounge-wear, you've likely expanded your fashion repertoire in ways that make you feel comfortable yet chic.

- Finding What Works for You: Every woman's pregnancy is unique, and so is her approach to maternity fashion. While some women feel empowered by fitted clothes that highlight their bump, others prefer looser, more relaxed styles. The beauty of maternity fashion is that there's no one-size-fits-all approach. You've found what works for you based on your body, your preferences, and your lifestyle, and this journey has likely deepened your understanding of how fashion can be both practical and personal.

Looking Ahead: How to Continue Dressing Comfortably and Stylishly Postpartum

As you transition from pregnancy to postpartum, your body will continue to change, and so will your wardrobe needs. Postpartum dressing presents its own set of challenges, but with the lessons you've learned from your maternity fashion journey, you'll be well-equipped to navigate this next phase with confidence.

1. The Fourth Trimester: Prioritizing Comfort and Functionality

The early postpartum period, often referred to as the "fourth trimester," is a time of healing, recovery, and adjustment. Your body will still be transitioning after childbirth, and comfort should remain a top priority during this time. However, just because you're prioritizing comfort doesn't mean you have to sacrifice style. Many of the pieces you wore during pregnancy—such as stretchy leggings, flowy tops, and maternity bras—can continue to serve you well in the postpartum phase.

- Nursing-Friendly Fashion: If you plan to breastfeed, you'll want to incorporate nursing-friendly clothing into your postpartum wardrobe. Look for tops and dresses with easy-access features like buttons, zippers, or wrap designs that make nursing convenient while still looking stylish. Nursing bras and tanks with built-in support can also provide comfort while ensuring you're ready for feedings.

- Loose and Comfortable Silhouettes: In the weeks and months following childbirth, you may still experience physical changes, including swelling, tenderness, and weight fluctuations. Loose-fitting, comfortable silhouettes like oversize sweaters, relaxed joggers, and flowy dresses will help you feel comfortable as your body continues to recover. Choose soft, breathable fabrics like cotton and jersey to keep you feeling cozy and supported.

- Luxe Lounge-wear and Robes: The postpartum period is a time when self-care is especially important. Treat yourself to luxurious Lounge-wear and soft robes that provide comfort and relaxation during those early days of bonding with your baby. Whether you're nursing, resting, or cuddling with your newborn, having cozy Lounge-wear will help you feel nurtured and cared for during this transition.

2. Embracing Postpartum Body Changes

Just as you adapted to your body's changes during pregnancy, the postpartum period will bring new shifts. It's important to be gentle with yourself during this time and to approach postpartum dressing with a mindset of self-compassion. Your body has just performed an incredible feat, and while it may take time to adjust to your new shape, there are plenty of ways to dress in a way that makes you feel confident and comfortable.

- Transitioning from Maternity to Regular Clothes: As your body heals and returns to its pre-pregnancy shape, you may find that some of your maternity clothes continue to serve you well, while others no longer fit. It's okay to take your time transitioning back to regular clothes—your comfort and confidence are the most important factors. Maternity leggings, stretchy dresses, and nursing tops are often versatile enough to be worn during the postpartum period, offering the support and flexibility you need as your body recovers.

- Investing in Postpartum Shapewear: Some women find that postpartum shape-wear helps them feel more supported and confident in the weeks after childbirth. Compression leggings, high-waited briefs, or belly bands can provide gentle support for your abdomen and back, making everyday activities more comfortable as your body heals. However, it's important to listen to your body and avoid wearing shape-wear that feels too restrictive.

- Rediscovering Your Style: As you adjust to life with a new baby, you'll also have the opportunity to rediscover your personal style. This might mean incorporating new trends, experimenting with different silhouettes, or simply finding joy in pieces that make you feel good. Remember that your postpartum wardrobe is an extension of your evolving identity, and you have the freedom to define what feels right for you.

Final Thoughts on Maternity Fashion and Comfort

Maternity fashion is about more than just finding clothes that fit—it's about embracing the changes your body goes through during pregnancy, celebrating your unique journey, and prioritizing your comfort and well-being. Throughout this process, you've likely discovered new ways to express yourself through fashion, whether that's by trying new trends, leaning into your personal style, or simply finding pieces that make you feel good in your skin.

1. The Power of Self-Expression Through Fashion

Fashion is a powerful form of self-expression, and this remains true during pregnancy. While maternity fashion may come with its own set of challenges, it also offers the opportunity to experiment, celebrate your body's changes, and honor your journey into motherhood. Whether you've embraced bold prints, athleisure, or minimalist looks, your maternity wardrobe reflects the beauty and strength of your evolving body.

2. Balancing Comfort and Style

One of the key lessons from your maternity fashion journey is that comfort and style are not mutually exclusive. Throughout your pregnancy, you've likely discovered that it's possible to feel both comfortable and stylish, whether you're wearing soft Lounge-wear at home or dressing up for a special occasion. This balance will continue to serve you well in the postpartum phase and beyond.

3. Confidence is Key

Ultimately, the most important aspect of maternity fashion is how it makes you feel. Confidence is key, and maternity fashion should empower you to embrace your body's changes with pride. Throughout your pregnancy journey, you've learned to adapt to your evolving shape and find clothing that not only fits but also makes you feel good about yourself. Whether you're flaunting your baby bump in a fitted dress or opting for a cozy, oversize sweater, the key is wearing what gives you confidence. Pregnancy is a time of transformation, and your fashion choices play a significant role in how you navigate these changes with self-assurance and grace.

Final Thoughts on Maternity Fashion and Comfort

As you reflect on your maternity fashion journey, it's clear that the right clothing can enhance both comfort and confidence. The goal of maternity fashion is to support you through each stage of pregnancy while allowing you to maintain your unique sense of style. From your first trimester to the postpartum period, your wardrobe has been a tool to help you feel at ease in your body, whether you're lounging at home or attending a special event.

1. Celebrating Your Journey

Your pregnancy journey is unlike anyone else's, and your maternity fashion choices have reflected that individuality. Each trimester brought new challenges and discoveries, and your wardrobe evolved to meet those needs. From adapting your pre-pregnancy wardrobe to investing in maternity essentials, you've learned to celebrate your body's incredible ability to grow and nurture life.

It's important to acknowledge that pregnancy isn't just about physical changes—it's an emotional journey, too. Maternity fashion can play a key role in how you experience these emotions. Whether it's finding a piece that boosts your confidence during a tough day or feeling the comfort of a perfectly fitted maternity bra, the clothes you choose can help you connect with yourself and your growing baby.

2. Looking Forward to Postpartum Style

As you move into the postpartum phase, your fashion journey will continue to evolve. Your body will keep changing, and your wardrobe will need to adapt once again. But with the lessons you've learned about prioritizing comfort, embracing your body, and staying true to your personal style, you'll be well-prepared to navigate this next chapter with ease.

Postpartum fashion doesn't have to be complicated. Many of the pieces that served you well during pregnancy—like stretchy leggings, comfortable dresses, and nursing-friendly tops—will continue to be wardrobe staples. As your body recovers and you find a new rhythm with your baby, you'll discover ways to blend comfort and style in your daily life.

3. Redefining Comfort and Style for the Long Term

Perhaps one of the biggest takeaways from your maternity fashion journey is the understanding that comfort and style are not opposing forces—they can work in harmony. This is a lesson that will extend beyond pregnancy and postpartum. Moving forward, you'll likely find that you continue to prioritize comfort in your everyday fashion choices, whether it's through the fabrics you wear, the cuts you choose, or the flexibility of your wardrobe.

Fashion is about feeling good in your skin, and that's especially important as you transition to motherhood. Maternity fashion has shown you that it's possible to look great while also honoring your body's needs. This understanding will serve you well as you continue to evolve your style for the long term.

Your maternity fashion journey is a deeply personal one, marked by growth, adaptation, and self-discovery. Throughout your pregnancy, you've learned to navigate the physical changes with grace and style, finding ways to blend comfort with fashion while celebrating your body's remarkable transformation.

As you reflect on this journey, remember that maternity fashion is about more than just clothes—it's about honoring the profound experience of becoming a mother. Your wardrobe has been a source of empowerment, helping you feel confident, comfortable, and true to yourself at every stage of pregnancy.

As you move forward into postpartum and beyond, continue to embrace the lessons you've learned about comfort, confidence, and self-expression. Your body will keep changing, and your style will evolve with it. But with the tools and insights you've gained from your maternity fashion journey, you'll be well-equipped to dress in a way that reflects your unique identity and makes you feel beautiful, inside and out.

Your maternity fashion journey has been a testament to your ability to adapt, to celebrate your body, and to find joy in the clothes you wear. Carry those lessons with you as you step into motherhood, confident in the knowledge that you can continue to look and feel your best, no matter where life takes you next.